Do
Timberline

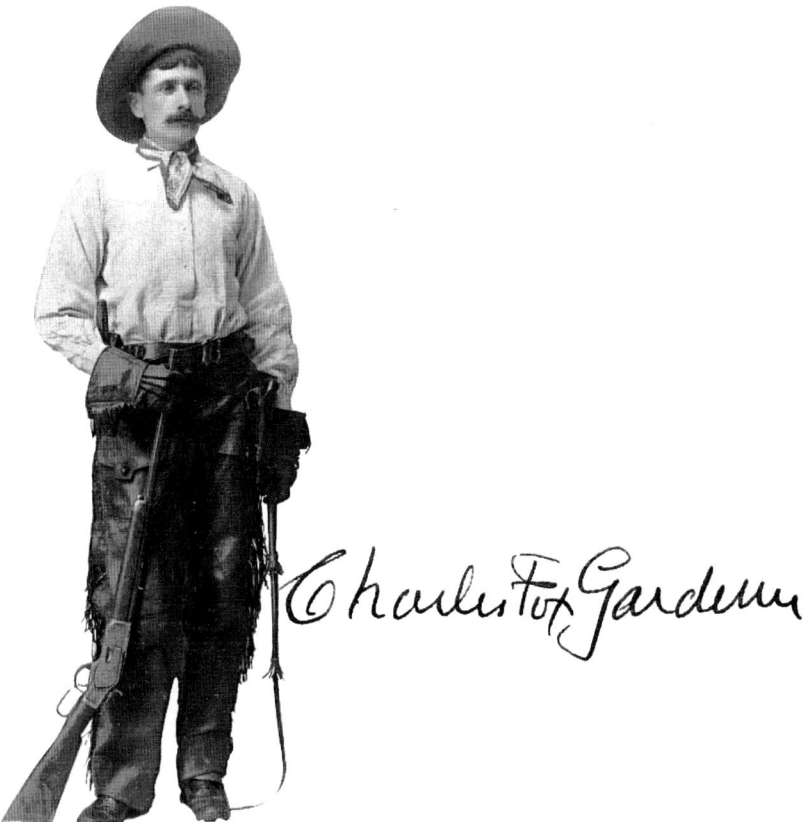

Charles Fox Gardenn

Pikes Peak Regional History Symposium
Sponsored by
Special Collections, Pikes Peak Library District
Friends of the Pikes Peak Library District
Pikes Peak Library District Foundation
Colorado Springs Pioneers Museum

In Partnership With
Evergreen Cemetery
Historic Preservation Alliance
McAllister House Museum
Pikes Peak Community College
Pikes Peak Posse of the Westerners
United States Air Force Academy
University of Colorado, Colorado Springs
Western Museum of Mining and Industry

Endorsed by

Project Director
Chris Nicholl

Pikes Peak Regional History Symposium Committee
Chris Nicholl, Co-Chair
Calvin P. Otto, Co-Chair

Steve Antonuccio	*Carol Kennis*
Tim Blevins	*Ingrid McDonald*
David Carroll	*Michael Olsen*
Dennis Daily	*Judith Rice Jones*
Beverly Diehl	*Mary Elizabeth Ruwell*
Dolores Fowler	*Kathy Sturdevant*
Barbara Gately	*Nancy Thaler*
Lynn A. Gilfillan-Morton	*Dee Vazquez*
Dianne Hartshorn	*Amy Ziegler*

Doctor at Timberline

True Tales, Travails, and Triumphs of a Pioneer Colorado Physician

by

Charles Fox Gardiner, M.D.

*Lavishly Illustrated with
Etchings, Engravings and Drawings
from Pikes Peak Library District
Special Collections*

Artfully Designed by Nancy Thaler

Published by

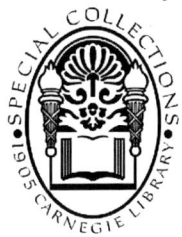

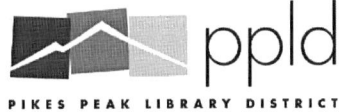

Doctor at Timberline: True Tales, Travails and Triumphs of a Pioneer Colorado Physician

Special contents © 2008 Pikes Peak Library District.

ISBN: 978-1-56735-254-2
Library of Congress Control Number: 2007937114
Printed in the United States.

All rights reserved.

This publication was made possible by private funds.

Originally published: Caldwell, Id.: The Caxton Printers, Ltd., © 1938. Reprinted with permission. New foreword, illustrations and afterword added. Includes bibliographical references.

For purchasing information, contact:
Clausen Books
2131 North Weber Street
Colorado Springs, Colorado 80907
tel: (719) 471-5884, toll free: (888)-412-7717
http://www.clausenbooks.com

About Pikes Peak Library District

Pikes Peak Library District (PPLD) is a nationally recognized system of public libraries serving a population of more than 500,000 in El Paso County, Colorado. With twelve facilities and two bookmobiles, PPLD responds to the unique needs of individual neighborhoods and the community at large. PPLD has an employee base of four hundred full and part-time staff, and utilizes roughly twelve hundred volunteers. It strives to reach all members of the community, providing free and equitable access to information and an avenue for personal and community enrichment.

PPLD is currently rated ninth among library systems its size in the country. Volume of circulations, number of visits, and hours of access contribute to the ranking. PPLD is also recognized for its commitment to diversity, its quality programming, and its excellent customer service.

Board of Trustees 2008

Robert J. Hilbert, President

John Wilson, Vice President

Calvin P. Otto, Secretary

Jill Gaebler

Aje Sakamoto

Katherine Spicer

Lynne Telford

Executive Director

Paula J. Miller

Regional History Series Editorial Committee

Tim Blevins
Dennis Daily
Chris Nicholl
Calvin P. Otto

Principal Series Consultant

Calvin P. Otto

Regional History Series

Currently In Print

The Colorado Labor Wars: Cripple Creek 1903–1904, A Centennial Commemoration

"To Spare No Pains": Zebulon Montgomery Pike and His 1806-1807 Southwest Expedition

Forthcoming

Extraordinary Women of the Rocky Mountain West

Legends, Labors & Loves: William Jackson Palmer, 1836–1909

Contents

Foreword • iii
Sources of Illustrations • v
Introduction • ix
Gardiner Letter • xxix
Preface • 3
A Tenderfoot Doctor on Ski and Bronco • 7
First Aid Above Timberline • 28
My Dream Horse • 43
The Widow's Herd • 55
My Tenderfoot • 65
A Tenderfoot Sheriff • 78
A Fourth of July in Cowtown • 96
A Hoodoo Trip • 106
A Tumor Clinic • 116
My Dog Czar • 120
Rough Surgery • 134
Coyote Basin • 145
A Storm Baby • 158
Mule Surgery • 166
A Cutting Affair • 170
"Ranch Jumping" • 183
"Jim" • 198
Some Hard Riding • 206
Lawless Justice • 216
Joe Bush and His Ride • 228

Acknowledgments

The Editorial Committee is indebted to the original publisher of Charles Fox Gardiner's *Doctor at Timberline*, Caxton Printers Ltd. of Caldwell, Idaho, for recognizing the significance of Dr. Gardiner's work when it was first released in 1938. We thank them, too, for consenting to our republishing this book as a primer to our 2008 Pikes Peak Regional History Symposium, *Doctors, Disease and Dying in the Pikes Peak Region*.

This edition was produced by the efforts of the staff in Special Collections, Pikes Peak Library District. An original *Timberline* was digitally scanned and converted to text by photodigitization expert Nina Kuberski. In addition to proofreading and design work, Photo Curator Nancy Thaler did a wonderful job researching, selecting and placing illustrations from publications contemporary to Dr. Gardiner's experiences in Colorado.

Our grateful thanks also go to Sydne Dean, PPLD's Associate Director for Public Services, whose constant encouragement and measured advice have been fundamental to every successful Special Collections endeavor.

We greatly appreciate the support that Colorado Humanities has provided for our annual Pikes Peak Regional History Symposia and for its endorsement of this Regional History Series publication.

Additionally, we wish to recognize John Stansfield, a storyteller and writer based in Larkspur, Colorado, who has portrayed Charles Fox Gardiner and told the *Timberline* stories to eager audiences for several years.

Lastly, we feel it proper to acknowledge Dr. Charles Fox Gardiner, as well as the woman to whom he dedicated his book seventy years ago—"To my dear friend and patient, Albertine C. Wales, whose unselfish encouragement and advice have made this book possible." Our hats off to both of them.

The Editorial Committee

Foreword

One can imagine the young Charles Fox Gardiner devouring every word describing the wild American West in the dime novels of the time. As a boy, he must have read these frontier tales during the late 1860s in the parlor of his New York City home. His position in society, education and chosen profession could easily have provided him a life of comfort with all of the amenities of wealth and privilege. Instead, the 25-year-old doctor set out to experience the Western Slope of Colorado's Rocky Mountains in January 1883.

It is not difficult to admire the backbone it must have required for Gardiner to travel to one of the most geographically isolated, questionably civilized, and just plain dangerous locations anywhere. Yet, when you read *Doctor at Timberline*, you will know his appetite for adventure did not go unsatisfied. Quite to the contrary, Gardiner's passion for this place is evident in the words he chooses to describe the incredibly beautiful country and the sometimes cruel, but awesome, climate. Keep a blanket handy— you will no doubt feel the bone-chilling cold as you read about his frigid trips on horseback and skis to help patients from prairies to mountaintops.

Doctor at Timberline is a collection of Gardiner's first-hand experiences as a physician in the new state of Colorado. He changed the names of the towns and the people in these true stories in a gentlemanly effort to conceal their identities. Many years have passed since Caxton Printers first published this book in 1938—and so, we are confident that revealing the true locations Gardiner describes will not arouse any offense. Crested Butte (*Silver Cup*), in Gunnison County, was the young coal-mining town where he first opened his medical practice in 1883. He married Emma "Daisy" Palmer Monteith in November 1884 and they set up housekeeping in Meeker (*Cowtown*), in Rio Blanco County. By 1887, the Gardiner family relocated to Colorado Springs, where he became internationally known for his theories on the treatment of tuberculosis.

Intended for a genteel readership of all ages, Gardiner leaves the "salty language" to the imagination of the reader by providing only a first letter from which there exist just a few words, in context, that can be fashioned. There are some words in this book that express the sometimes racist views of the times towards various ethnic groups. Rather than revise this book, it is reprinted as it was originally written. However, wonderful Frederic Remington and Charles Russell drawings have been added, and they beautifully illustrate and augment Gardiner's stirring narrative.

Some of Gardiner's stories explore provocative subjects that merit examination and discussion. Morality, ethics and honor (the "Code of the West") are juxtaposed with abuse, murder and lawlessness. These circumstances, paired with emotion, humor, self reflection, triumph, and regret, combine in his stories to form a picture of what life was really like in Colorado during the last quarter of the nineteenth century. Despite Colorado's natural beauty, life in the West just wasn't always that pretty.

There is scarcely a mention of Daisy, Gardiner's wife, or their two children, Raynor and Dorothy, anywhere in his book except in the story "My Dog Czar." In fact, not one of them is identified by name. Tragically, tuberculosis took Daisy's life in March 1893. She was buried in Evergreen Cemetery, Colorado Springs, in a plot where Charles Gardiner later joined her in July 1947. His second wife of fifty years, Fanny S. Anderson, died in June 1954—and was also interred in the same plot.

If there are only a few books you read more than once, I can guarantee *Doctor at Timberline* will make that list. Gardiner's vignettes of early Colorado come across as a friend or neighbor would tell them. It is, therefore, easy to read through all the stories—picturing the hard yet gorgeous terrain, getting to know the characters, anticipating their quirky (yet altogether real!) situations—and ending the book, wanting more. Grieve not!

Chris Nicholl, Local History Specialist in Pikes Peak Library District's Special Collections, has written an insightful introduction about Dr. Gardiner that provides a delightful taste of his life before and after the exploits he described in *Doctor at Timberline*. No doubt you will hunger to read Nicholl's complete interpretive essay about Gardiner in the forthcoming book in the Regional History Series, *Doctors, Disease and Dying in the Pikes Peak Region*.

It is our honor to reprint *Doctor at Timberline* in conjunction with PPLD's fifth annual Pikes Peak Regional History Symposium.

Paula J. Miller, Executive Director, PPLD

Tim Blevins, Manager, Special Collections, PPLD

Sources of Illustrations

Page:

Cover Composite illustration by Nancy Thaler, combining "Timberline Trees" by Harry L. Standley and portrait of Dr. Gardiner, ca. 1885.

ix Charles Fox Gardiner, 1898.

x Charles Fox Gardiner, ca. 1885.

xiv Billy Edwards, trading card, Mecca Cigarettes, n.d.

xvii Dr. Gardiner's home in Meeker, Colorado, 1884.

xix Dr. Gardiner and family at the cabin in Meeker, Colorado, n.d.

xxi Nordrach Ranch Sanatorium, ca. 1906.

xxiv Dr. and Mrs. Gardiner, ca. 1900.

xxiv Four generations of Gardiner family, 1942.

6 Map of Colorado by James Monteith, 1885.

8 "Colorado – Life in the Mining Districts." *Frank Leslie's Illustrated Newspaper*, June 7, 1879.

17 "Staking Claims," detail from "Adventures in the San Juans." *Harper's Weekly*, June 9, 1893.

19 "Snow-Shoeing 'A Mile A Minute,'" detail from "Adventures in the San Juans." *Harper's Weekly*, June 9, 1893.

21 Quarrel over card game, Frederic Remington. *Harper's Weekly*, April 23, 1887.

24 "The Recent Terrific Blizzards in the West," detail. *Frank Leslie's Illustrated Newspaper*, February 1, 1890.

30 "Mules Loaded with Winter Stores, Revenue Mines," detail from "Sketches in the Colorado Mining Districts, North America." *The Illustrated London News*, November 6, 1880.

31 "A Snow Slide in the Rocky Mountains." *Harper's Weekly*, February 17, 1883.

38 "An Awkward Corner," R. Caton Woodville, detail from "Hunting Wild Goats in the Rocky Mountains, North America." *The Illustrated London News*, November 27, 1886.

44 "Rawhide Rawlins' Horse," Charles Russell, n.d.

46	"Breaking Wild Horses," detail, Jerome Smith and Charles Russell. *Frank Leslie's Illustrated Newspaper*, May 18, 1889.
50	"Breaking Wild Horses," detail, Jerome Smith and Charles Russell. *Frank Leslie's Illustrated Newspaper*, May 18, 1889.
54	Ginger, R. H. Hall. From *Doctor at Timberline*, 1938.
58	Cutting a steer out of the herd, Frederic Remington. From *Ranch Life and the Hunting-Trail* by Theodore Roosevelt, 1888.
61	Cowboys guarding herd at night, Frenzeny and Tavernier. *Harper's Weekly*, March 28, 1874.
66	Stagecoach, Jerome H. Smith. *Frank Leslie's Illustrated Newspaper*, January 25, 1890.
68	"Invitation of the Tenderfoot," Charles Russell, n.d.
72	Colorado cowboys, W. A. Rogers. *Harper's Weekly*, October 6, 1883.
73	Post trader, Charles Russell, n.d.
79	Nevada stagecoach, H. F. Farny. *Harper's Weekly*, March 22, 1890.
84	Shooting walnuts, R. H. Hall. From *Doctor at Timberline*, 1938.
90	"Fight in the Street," Frederic Remington. *Century Magazine*, October 1888.
99	"Thanksgiving Dinner for the Ranch," detail, Frederic Remington. *Harper's Weekly*, November 24, 1888.
103	"Shooting Up Main Street," Paul Frenzeny. *Frank Leslie's Illustrated Newspaper*, January 14, 1882.
104	Mormon family, detail, Frenzeny and Tavernier. *Harper's Weekly*, January 2, 1875.
109	Indian Raid, C. S. Reinhart. *Harper's Weekly*, July 16, 1870.
112	"The Cow-boys of Colorado—Life in a Dug-out," W. A. Rogers. *Harper's Weekly*, November 18, 1882.
114	"Elk Horn Ranch Buildings," Frederic Remington. From *Ranch Life and the Hunting-Trail* by Theodore Roosevelt, 1888.
116	"Ejecting an Oklahoma Boomer," detail, T. de Thulstrap, based

Sources of Illustrations

on a sketch by Frederic Remington. *Harper's Weekly*, March 28, 1885.

121   Dog, W. M. Caro, detail from "Indian Boys Breaking a Pony." *Harper's Weekly*, May 2, 1874.

126   "It was nothing at all to climb this awful trail with Czar pulling me," R. H. Hall. From *Doctor at Timberline*, 1938.

130   Cavalry troop caught in a blizzard, detail, R. F. Zogbaum. *Harper's Weekly*, January 28, 1888.

134   "Miner's Cabin." *Supplement to Harper's Weekly*, January 19, 1889.

136   Packhorse, detail from photo of Charles Fox Gardiner and his horses, 1880. Courtesy of Mrs. W. D. Hemming.

142   "On Guard at Night," Frederic Remington. From *Ranch Life and the Hunting-Trail* by Theodore Roosevelt, 1888.

143   Rustlers caught in the act, Charles Russell, n.d.

148   "Pleasant Park." From "Glimpses of Colorado," March 15, 1873.

149   "Hard Trail," Frederic Remington. From *Ranch Life and the Hunting-Trail* by Theodore Roosevelt, 1888.

155   Ranch at Greeley, n.d.

160   Old-Time Cow Ranch, Charles Russell, n.d.

161   "I found a rope stretched from the corral to the house," R. H. Hall. From *Doctor at Timberline*, 1938.

166   "Calling for the Relays," Frenzeny and Tavernier. *Harper's Weekly*, July 4, 1874.

172   Woman attacked. *The Illustrated Police News*, ca. 1875.

178   "Trial Scene in Colorado Mining Town," Alfred Mitchell. *Frank Leslie's Illustrated Newspaper*, November 27, 1887.

179   Trial in Leavenworth, Kansas, 1857.

184   "Elk Horn Ranch Buildings," Frederic Remington. From *Ranch Life and the Hunting-Trail* by Theodore Roosevelt, 1888.

192   "Taking the Morning 'Slumgullion,'" detail, Frenzeny and Tavernier. *Harper's Weekly*, July 4, 1874.

195	"Vigilante Justice," Hyde. *Frank Leslie's Illustrated Newspaper*, November 12, 1881.
196	"Territorial Indignation Meeting," J. W. Orr, ca. 1857.
200	"Colorado—The Mining Town Rico," detail, ca. 1881.
202	1880s Cowboy, based on photo by C. D. Kirkland. *Frank Leslie's Illustrated Newspaper*, April 9, 1887.
207	Army scout, detail, T. de Thulstrup. *Harper's Weekly*, August 1, 1885.
212	Fight in saloon, Frederic Remington. In *Ranch Life and the Hunting-Trail* by Theodore Roosevelt, 1888.
215	"The Travaux Pony," detail, Frederic Remington. From "Some American Riders" by Theo. A. Dodge, in *Harper's Monthly*, May 1891.
220	In a Rocky Mountain hotel dining room, A. C. Redwood, detail from a sketch by Alfred Mitchell. *Harper's Weekly*, August 30, 1887.
224	"'Hands Up!' The Capture of Finnegan," Frederic Remington. In *Ranch Life and the Hunting-Trail* by Theodore Roosevelt, 1888.
230	"Calling the Night Guard," Frenzeny and Tavernier, ca. 1875.
235	"A Spanish-Californian Type." From "Life in California Before the Gold Discovery" in *Century Magazine*, December 1890.
241	"The Fandango," George Wharton Edwards. From "Pioneer Spanish Families in California," [*Century Magazine?*], 1891.
246	"Dragging a bull's hide over a prairie fire in Northern Texas," detail, Frederic Remington. *Harper's Weekly*, October 27, 1888.

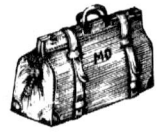

Introduction

The Trials and Tribulations of a Hinterland Physician of Pioneer Days, or, "Damn it, I Wanted to be Ninety"

by Chris Nicholl

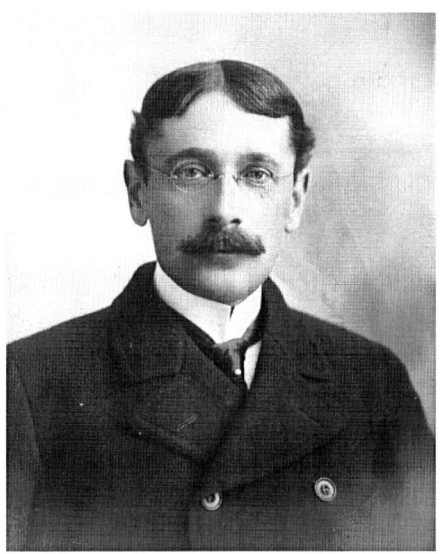

Dr. Charles Fox Gardiner, 1898. *Photograph from Special Collections, Pikes Peak Library District.*

Of the year's bumper crop of books by physicians, this is the most exciting.

DOCTOR AT TIMBERLINE by Charles Fox Gardiner

If any one should buy this book and not like it, I shall either eat the book or buy it from him at the exact price he paid for it. There is not a dull page in the entire work. . . . My hat is off to the doctor who wrote it. William Lyon Phelps[1]

  The advertisement quoted above illustrates the critical acclaim awarded Charles Fox Gardiner's book, *Doctor at Timberline*, following its 1938 publication. The book is a compilation of short, colorful and often amusing anecdotes detailing Gardiner's adventures as a "tenderfoot" physician in Colorado in the mid-1880s.

A well-educated man from a prestigious Eastern family, Gardiner was both participant and sensitive observer of Colorado's mining and ranching settlement as well as an astute chronicler of human frailty and strength. In his stories, Gardiner recorded the "life of hardship and bravely faced dangers"of the silver miners he met in the snow-covered mountains at Crested Butte in Gunnison County. Moving on to the cow town of Meeker in Rio Blanco County, he was the only physician in that "wild unsettled region" for a hundred miles around. Traveling by skis, horseback, or buggy, Gardiner treated the miners and ranchers who came from all classes, and he described their varying degrees of morality and character.

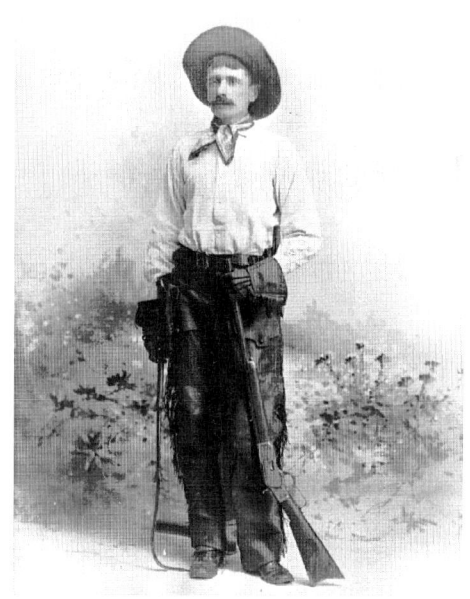

Charles Fox Gardiner in a studio portrait showing his "western" clothes, ca. 1885. *Photograph from Special Collections, Pikes Peak Library District.*

Some fifty years later, by then a retired Colorado Springs physician, Gardiner wrote up his case notes. He planned to leave the manuscript of his pioneering adventures to his children. Encouraged by others who recognized his memoirs as a significant historical document, he published his book.[2] Marketed as a "true picture" of the early days of the west, the book was an immediate hit and a "Book of the Month Club" recommendation. In 1940, William Lyon Phelps, a famous literary critic and Yale University professor whose quote opens this essay, included it among the year's best books, along with titles by some of the era's finest writers such as Carl Sandburg and Somerset Maugham. The book was reissued in 1939, 1940, and 1946, including a London edition. Copies remain in public libraries and in university, research, and medical school libraries throughout the English-speaking world.[3]

As one reviewer described it, *Doctor at Timberline* is "a first-hand reflection of the western gold camp days" recalled by a physician whose "patients were miners and cowboys and murderers and just plain folks."[4] The book is filled with characters and events drawn large—so much so that Gardiner remarked,

> Some folks accuse me of stretching truth to the breaking point in my autobiography, but the fact is I omitted many things because I believed they would be looked upon as fabrications. I had to hold a tight rein on truth, for fear it would not be believed. And even then I seem to have strained the credulity of some readers.[5]

Gardiner's memoirs are a testament to twenty-first-century readers of the nearly unbelievable dangers and unbearable adversity faced by the founding mothers and fathers of the American West. The stories recount how Colorado's pioneers adjusted to the unsettled time and place and shaped it with courage, optimism, quick-witted grit, chivalrous kindness, and cruel humor, with a bit of homicide and genocide along the way.

Reading Gardiner's absorbing account in the first decade of the twenty-first century, roughly one hundred twenty years after the events, offers the present-day Colorado audience a twofold view of the past: it provides us the opportunity to learn of our founding through the author's personal reflections on the developing west; and, by examining the book's reviews and its popular acclaim upon its first appearance seventy years ago, we can make assumptions about the sensibilities of the era in which it was published.

In his anecdotes, Gardiner speaks of the origins of modern-day Coloradoans. The west's settlers immigrated from around the nation, Europe and Asia. He describes a time and place, devoid of ideas of political correctness, and offering something to offend the sensibilities of everyone through slurs and pejorative nicknames.

There is a Chinese cook on one ranch and a "darky" cook, Black Charlie, on another. There are Arizona Bill and Frenchy, two murderous desperados. We meet Shorty, Fatty Murphy the blacksmith, and Slim Tex. There is a "good-natured fat Jew," a traveling whisky merchant. We encounter Swedes from Canada and Norwegians, who fabricated custom-designed "snowshoes" and introduced skiing to Crested Butte for transportation and recreation, thus establishing the foundations of the Colorado ski industry.[6] There is Dutch Charlie, and Scotty the shoemaker, who, attired in full Highland costume, plays a funeral dirge on his bagpipe. We meet Mr. Collins from Boston who "appeared and acted like a gentleman," and the Wilson brothers, John and Tom, Ohio natives who represent the intrepid pioneer miners of Colorado's past and present lucrative mining industry.[7] They were "hardy and reckless men . . . skillful, strong and brave . . ." who ". . . would endure any danger or hardship if they saw a chance of grasping a fortune from fate." There were "half-breeds," the despised offspring of Anglos and American Indians and there are "squaws," a common but cruel-sounding word for American Indian women. We meet a "Mormon from a new settlement of Latter-day Saints . . . all whiskers, and very dirty, ignorant, and fanatical, with a mean, sullen temper." There is Mex Joe the barkeep, and references to Mexicans as "greasers."

The monikers, whether denoting ethnic or national origin or descriptive of body type or ideology, offer present-day readers insight into the range of immigrants who peopled early Colorado. Today, some of the terms, ordinary in the 1880s, are unacceptably racist and cruel; and as the names passed unremarked in the original reviews, they reveal the social acceptance of such demeaning stereotypes in the literature of the late 1930s.

Much of Gardiner's account is devoted to descriptions of ordinary people going about their lives. When he experienced

Introduction

his adventures, Gardiner was likely unaware that he was living among, treating, and describing the quintessential American character, the cowboy. Gardiner found much to admire in the virtues and habits of the cowboys he treated and befriended in and around the Colorado boomtowns. In scattered passages throughout his book, Gardiner defines the various components of a "cowboy code" that taken together create the mythic image of the cowboys and cattlemen that permeates popular culture in tales of the west, whether in movies, television or novels—"a coarse violent man, but a very gallant gentleman."

Charles Fox Gardiner was born on October 12, 1857, in New York City and died in Colorado Springs on July 31, 1947. The sickly, only child of a wealthy businessman, Gardiner grew up in a world of uncommon privilege that he described as "well-off without wealth."[8] The Gardiner family, although owning a home in Yonkers, spent winters at the prestigious Fifth Avenue Hotel, the latest thing in accommodations in 1862. By age five, Charles lived a heady, cultivated life. He noted,

> I was an only child and spoiled pretty badly. Long before I had long trousers I led a man-of-the-world life when I should have been in school. I went everywhere, saw everything, sat up late and was as wise to all the sin and scandal of a big city as any adult.[9]

Standing five feet seven inches tall and weighing in at only one hundred ten pounds, Gardiner's daughter, Dorothy Hemming, remembered him as "very light, slender and very, very full of pep."[10] Made self-conscious by his small stature and youthful infirmities, Gardiner wrestled with low self-esteem. To boost his confidence and his physique, he went daily to a gymnasium, meeting and training with the era's respected athletes. There he benefited from the guidance of a famous physiologist, Austin Flint, as a sort of personal trainer.[11] Barnum's circus stars taught him gymnastics. Under the tutelage of the world-famous prizefighter, Billy Edwards, Gardiner, known as "Spider," won the title of

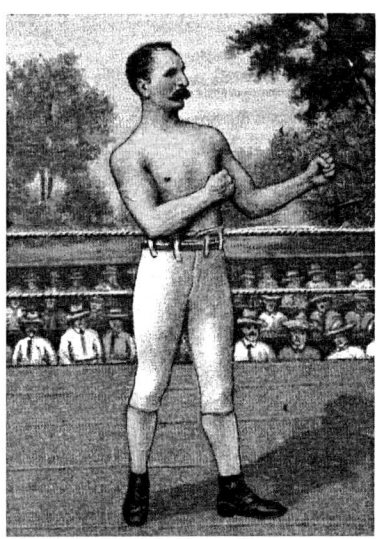

Billy Edwards (1844 – ca. 1908), known as "the pugilistic marvel of his age," was one of the most famous lightweight boxers of his time. Standing five feet four and five-eighths inches tall and weighing one hundred and twenty-six pounds, Edwards probably met and beat more men than any fighter of his size and weight, all with bare knuckles.
Trading card: Mecca Cigarettes "Champion Athlete & Champion Series.

New York State Featherweight Amateur Boxing Champion.[12] Along the way, he designed and built his own canoe, took long trips (stopping at posh resorts around Long Island, including his ancestral home, Gardiner's Island), and, after wrecking his craft, won another in a canoeing competition against a field of eighteen husky competitors.[13] He took up long distance running to build his endurance and spent days hiking the mountains of upstate New York, honing his wilderness survival skills.

Some biographical accounts describe him as a former consumptive who had come to Colorado to regain his health.[14] If true, that might explain his interest in the relationship between climate and tuberculosis, the field of medicine in which he later specialized. Although regularly suffering blinding migraine headaches, Gardiner makes no reference to having consumption. Instead he wrote, "gradually, by years of practice, [I] hardened my thin, frail body so that, although I was not big and strong, I was very active and could tire out many of my stronger friends." In Colorado his fit body and rigorous lifestyle brought him through the onerous hardships of travel in the snowbound mountains and on the torturous horseback rides in the deserts and canyons around Meeker.

Along with his determination to overcome his innate physical limitations, Gardiner pursued other interests leading to his careers as a frontier physician and finally as the author of a best-selling

Introduction

autobiography. Writing of his youth, Gardiner confessed, "I always had a great desire to be an explorer. I read all the books I could find on the subject, and men who went to the unknown parts of the earth were my heroes." From his reading, he imagined himself the hero in some wild, untamed place and the seeds of heroic imagery flourished in his western adventures.

Gardiner's unpublished accounts reveal that very early on he had a medical bent and an adventurous spirit. Before he turned twelve years old, Charles had visited the capitals of the western world: London, Edinburgh, Amsterdam, Rotterdam, Berlin, Dresden, Munich, Paris, Berne, Venice, Naples and Rome. It was in Paris during that European tour with his parents that he developed his fascination with medicine and healing. Seeing firsthand the bloody Franco–Prussian War [July 1870-May 1871], he recalled the sounds of guns near Paris, the despair of the beaten French, and he said,

> I was not afraid, but only wanted to do something. Across the street just back of our hotel a small hospital was established, a kind of clearing station for the wounded from the forts outside Paris. I crowded among the people to see the ambulances unload the wounded. I felt a strange desire to go right among them and help.

The shy and delicate-looking young boy was told that children were not allowed, but he refused to back away. After he helped save the wounded son of a French military officer from a falling stretcher, the grateful man gave the small American boy the run of the hospital, where he carried water and dressings and occasionally, to his delight, held an arm or a leg during an amputation.[15]

At eighteen, with no regular education or training for any useful work, he began learning the rudiments of the business world under the tutelage of a cultivated, kindly silk importer, a friend of his father. However, his tasks of copying letters, running errands and collecting bills were secondary to his interest in comparative anatomy. He began to dissect cats, drawing and coloring charts of their muscles, nerves and blood vessels, during working hours and in the absence of his employer. His business education abruptly ended when he forgot to dispose of one of his specimens, leaving it to be discovered by his boss, along with his meticulously-rendered anatomy charts.

His tolerant employer contacted a surgeon friend who recognized Charles for the natural doctor that he was. The silk merchant encouraged Charles' father to allow him to study medicine. A week later he "was sitting on the hard benches of the College of Physicians and Surgeons . . . and working sixteen hours a day with delight, a work [he] loved, and the hated business was left for ever."[16]

Following some starts and stops, Gardiner ultimately earned an M.D. from the Bellevue Hospital Medical College; he interned at a charity hospital, worked as a prison surgeon, and with the ambulance service of a New York hospital.[17]

By 1882, Gardiner was positioned to live out the daring life he had dreamed of. He was as physically fit as he could be, he possessed the wilderness survival skills to realize his ambition of western adventure, he was educated and experienced as a physician, and he imagined for himself a heroic self-image.

On a cold January day of 1883, Gardiner arrived in snowbound Crested Butte, expecting to stay in Colorado for a year or so to experience firsthand "some wild place."[18]

The community of around twelve hundred people already had two trusted physicians,[19] and Gardiner's business was slow to take off. But, after proving his mettle by undertaking a perilous house call above timberline, risking his own life to treat an injured miner, Gardiner was assured an income. He was hired as the surgeon for the Colorado Coal and Iron Company that owned many of the region's coal mines and coke manufacturers.[20]

An 1883 newspaper article promoting the region and describing the abundant game, magnificent beauty and excellent accommodations in Gunnison County helps to explain why a privileged youth, even with a prestigious pedigree such as Gardiner's, might not only venture west but make it his home. And Gardiner often expressed his never-ending awe of Colorado's sublime beauty.

Introduction

Before traveling to Colorado, Gardiner was betrothed to Emma "Daisy" Monteith, the daughter of a famous eastern geographer, James Monteith. Daisy, seemingly with a streak of audacity as bold as Charles', came west. On November 20, 1884, the young couple was married at Grace Episcopal Church in Colorado Springs. Family lore claimed that Daisy's father objected to her living in the rough and rowdy mining camp, so Charles settled in the nascent cattle town of Meeker where things were quieter;[21] however, the record suggests otherwise. Departing from the Antlers Hotel the day following their nuptials, the Gardiners boarded the 10:45 a.m. Denver & Rio Grande train bound for Crested Butte,[22] where the June 1, 1885, Colorado census reveals that they were living. Four men, described as "batching," were also enumerated at their household—two silver miners (one from Canada, another from Iowa), a coal miner from England, and a laborer from Kentucky.[23] For Daisy, whose childhood home in New York City had included three or four servants,[24] camp life in a household

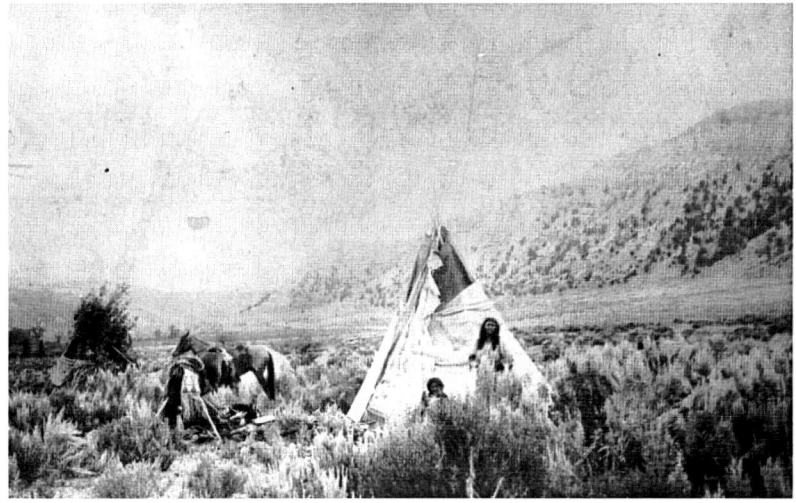

Utes often camped near Dr. Gardiner's home in Meeker. His admiration of their tipi design and lifestyle including fresh air and sunshine inspired his fresh air tuberculosis treatment and led to his design of the "Gardiner Tent." This photo was taken behind Dr. Gardiner's home in Meeker in 1884. *Photograph from Special Collections, Pikes Peak Library District, courtesy of Mrs. W. D. Hemming.*

with four laboring bachelors must have seemed far removed from her upbringing as the youngest daughter of a prominent Easterner.

By the fall of 1885, according to Jack Schaefer's biographical account, *Heroes without Glory*, the Gardiners were living in Meeker, awaiting the birth of their first child. Schaefer wrote that while Daisy had adapted to life in the "raw rough West and had taken the change in stride and never complained overmuch about being so far from civilization . . . she might need better care than [Charles] could give her or get for her in Meeker."[25] Escaping the doctor's grueling work schedule, the Gardiners traveled by buckboard some three hundred miles from Meeker to Colorado Springs. Both Schaefer and the Gardiner's daughter, Dorothy Hemming, described the journey as a romantic getaway for the young newlyweds, a six-day jolly jaunt of camping in the mountains and sleeping underneath the wagon, taken just two weeks before the birth of their son, Raynor.[26]

Schaefer's reasoning for the Gardiners' lengthy journey — in an open buckboard, during Colorado's unpredictable fall weather and when the physician husband recorded delivering babies in breathtakingly dangerous situations — could be correct. However, as Daisy's family visited Colorado Springs for extended times, perhaps she longed to be near her family for the birth of her first child.[27] After six weeks of town life, the Gardiners returned to Meeker with their infant son.

Meeker pioneer, Maggie Henry Cassidy, recalled that around 1885, there was little to hold a family there — no schools or churches, just a post office and the Meeker Hotel.[28] According to the family story, the Gardiners moved to Colorado Springs, seeking better educational opportunities for their young son.

As the child was but two years old, perhaps the move was also prompted by other factors, such as the isolation of frontier life. Built a quarter mile from town, primarily to escape the around-the-clock revelry of Meeker's saloons, Gardiner's cabin elicited fond memories. Reached by a little bridge crossing over a nearby stream, it was nestled in a meadow that offered a pleasant view.

Introduction

He recalled an evening, when contemplating a time with his books, he gazed through his cabin window, enjoying a view of soft snow falling and the glimmering lights from nearby Meeker:

> My room looked very cozy and comfortable with soft easy chairs, rugs, a German student lamp on the table, a shelf of books; and my open fire very bright and warm as it threw shadows among the deer heads on the wall and was reflected from my rifles in a rack below them.

Writing of that scene some fifty years later, his little home appeared romantic. But the reality of the primitive conditions in which he and his family lived is revealed in a family portrait. Flanked by two dogs, the little family posed at the front of a log cabin. While the ell-shaped house appears soundly built, with windows charmingly draped by tied back curtains, the landscape appears dreary, barren and isolated. Gardiner's passage in which he articulated his sick fear for the safety of his undefended wife and baby when rumors circulated of a Ute uprising perhaps contributed to their move. Perhaps, too, it was the far-flung house calls that kept him away from his little family for extended

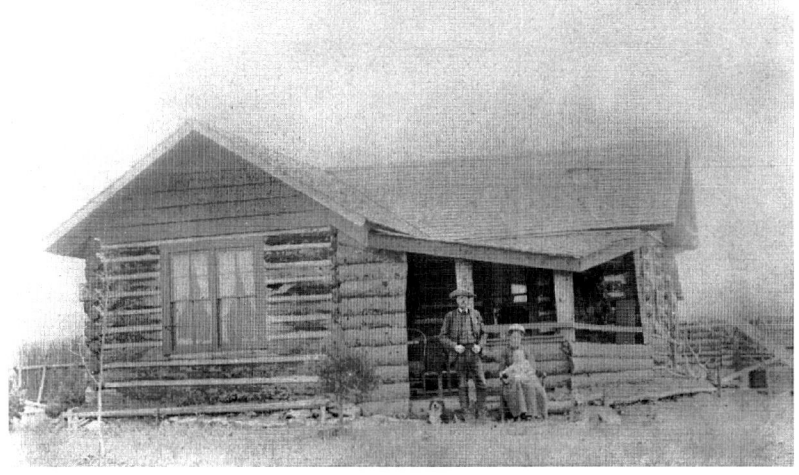

This undated photo shows Dr. Charles Fox Gardiner and his family at their cabin in Meeker, Colorado. *Photograph from Special Collections, Pikes Peak Library District.*

periods of time that motivated Charles and Daisy to relocate. Whatever the reason, Charles filed his medical license with the El Paso County Clerk in September 1887.[29] In the 1888 *Colorado Springs City Directory*, the Gardiners were residing at 224 East Pikes Peak Avenue where Charles was also practicing medicine.[30] Their daughter Dorothy arrived in December 1891.

Daisy died in March 1893 at age thirty, "after a lingering illness of many months."[31] It was said that she had contracted tuberculosis from her sister, Lillian, who had moved west seeking a cure. Devastated, Gardiner journeyed back to Meeker alone, where he selected and returned with the perfect piece of granite that marks her burial place at Evergreen Cemetery.[32] Dorothy, only fifteen months old when her mother died, recalled that her father "broke down completely and had to go back to a sanatorium in New York to get well." In his young daughter's memory, Gardiner's recovery required several years. She remembered that two "old maids, Quaker ladies," wrote to her father, suggesting they should move into his house to care for his children, arguing that the Irish servants were doing a poor job of it. Gardiner was, "of course . . . simply delighted" and the ladies, Dorothy thought, took care of his children "until he married again."[33] Gardiner married Fannie S. Anderson in April 1897, in "a quiet ceremony," so described in *Facts* Magazine, a sort of nineteenth-century tabloid filled with bits of social news and gossip about the city's elite.[34]

In Colorado Springs, Gardiner practiced medicine for nearly fifty years. Like others of his local colleagues, the doctor wore many hats.[35] He was a general practitioner and a tuberculosis specialist, a town booster, a teacher, a scientific researcher, and an author. He was a sanatorium founder and administrator, and he was the inventor of the Gardiner Tent, a popular treatment model that forced consumptives to live in a nearly outdoor setting all the year around. Through presenting his research to meetings of state and national medical associations, Gardiner quickly built his reputation as an expert in the study and treatment of tuberculosis. In 1892 he published "Immunity from Phthisis [tuberculosis] as affected by altitude in Colorado."

Introduction

Gardiner was an early member and president of the El Paso County Medical Society, founded in 1879. He was a member of the Colorado College Scientific Society, established in 1890 for "discussion of recent scientific results, the promotion among its members of scientific inquiry and investigation and the publication of the more important papers read at its meetings," and he served as a lecturer at the Colorado College from 1894–1895.[36] By 1897, Gardiner was traveling to national medical association meetings in the east, and was collaborating with other physicians on editing *The Climatologist*, a journal dedicated to the treatment and study of consumption. In collaboration with the city's Chamber of Commerce as a town booster, in 1898 Gardiner published *The Colorado Springs Region as a Health and Pleasure Resort*. Throughout the following decades he touted Colorado's palliative climate for consumptives in more than a dozen published papers, boosting the economies of the Colorado Springs region and its medical community.[37]

Dr. Gardiner believed that fresh air and sunshine were the major components in treating tuberculosis and he thought that a tent was the closest thing to living outside. Applying his theories to the treatment of tuberculosis, Gardiner spent ten years

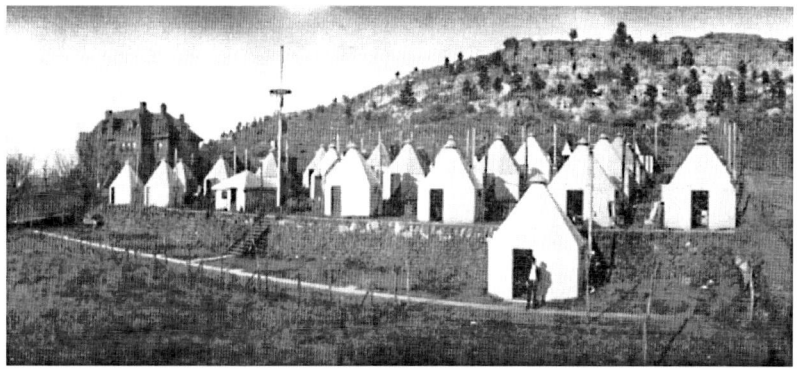

Dr. John E. White established the Nordrach Ranch Sanatorium at Austin Bluffs near Colorado Springs in 1901. Named and patterned after a successful German sanatorium that emphasized fresh air, disciplined gluttony, and restricted physical activity, it contained more than fifty Gardiner tents plus several rooms in the existing stone house for critically ill patients. *Photograph ca. 1906, from Special Collections, Pikes Peak Library District.*

developing his "sanatory" tent. He arranged with the Colorado Springs Tent and Awning Company to manufacture it. The tent was made of "very heavy duck" stretched over a wood frame, measuring sixteen feet in diameter. The tent, like the octagonal Ute tipi, was open at the top and had fresh air inlets at the base. A wood or coal stove heated it. The tent became very popular and along with its other form, a wooden tipi-shaped structure, it was the model of, and virtually synonymous, with the open-air therapy of tuberculosis.[38]

Gardiner's fresh air therapy caught on. Besides the tent cities such as the Modern Woodman of America sanatorium, many of the Victorian-era houses that line the North End of downtown Colorado Springs reveal the architectural influence of Gardiner and other physicians who, without antibiotics to treat tuberculosis, believed that screened porches, lots of sunshine, and adequate fresh air would benefit the consumptive. Throughout the region, "open-air sleeping porches and balconies began sprouting from the upper stories of houses and outside the windows of hospitals." Some physicians, such as Gerald Webb, who thought Gardiner a bit fanatical in his devotion to fresh air treatment, tried sleeping in a fresh air porch on a few wintry nights, and agreed that upon waking he felt "wonderfully fit."[39]

By 1923, Drs. Gardiner and Webb, both well-known specialists in their field, jointly published a statistical study of how altitude affected the mortality rate in tuberculosis. In May 1924, Webb organized the nonprofit Colorado Foundation for Research in Tuberculosis of which Dr. Gardiner was an associate member. That foundation, renamed the Webb-Waring Lung Institute at the University of Colorado, continues today for the research and treatment of lung disease.[40]

Charles Fox Gardiner was a great storyteller. His anecdotes of pioneer days in the mining and ranching regions of Colorado's Western Slope inform a new audience of the trials and travails of early-day settlers, and his stories transmit little life lessons to the observant reader. Gardiner, always owning his foibles and weaknesses, offered up one of life's most valuable lessons when he told of a lynch mob of around one hundred men threatening

Introduction

to hang a man. A courageous man dampened the crowd's rage. Gardiner recalled, "I have always wished that I had not waited but had been first [to face down the mob]." Gardiner's admission, some fifty years after the fact, that he once feared to stand up for a moral principle in spite of popular opposition, haunted him for life.

In reading and digesting Gardiner's stories, we notice that our intrepid and intelligent author offered not only life lessons, but he prepared a feast of questions for us to ponder. Who were we at the beginning? Who are we now? How far have we come? Or have we come far at all? And, of greater importance, where are we going and who will we become?

What appears at first glance to be a winsome memoir of an aged man, romanticized by the passing of time, in fact becomes a starting point for examination of our contemporary identity as Americans and as westerners; perhaps, upon reflection of Gardiner's heroic themes and mythic images that overlay multiple subtexts with their issues of racism, domestic and community violence, imperialism and genocide, sacrifice and redemption, we will reflect upon redefining our national purpose.

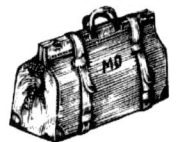

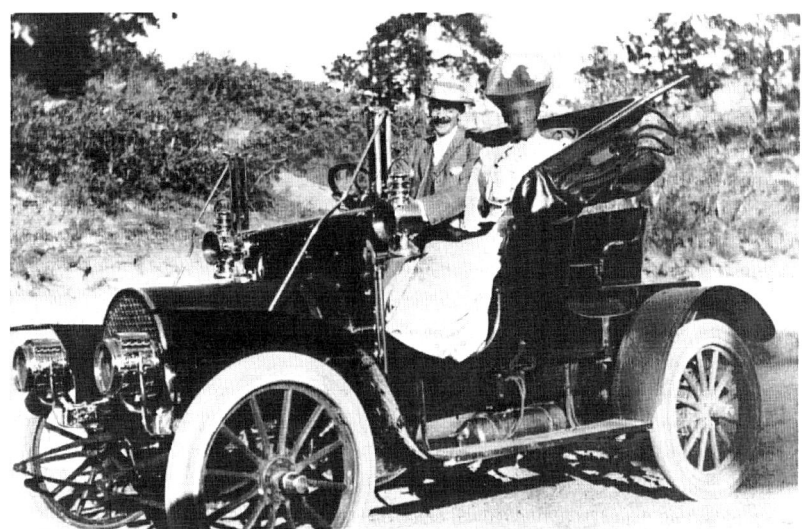

Dr. and Mrs. Gardiner, ca. 1900. *Photograph from Special Collections, Pikes Peak Library District.*

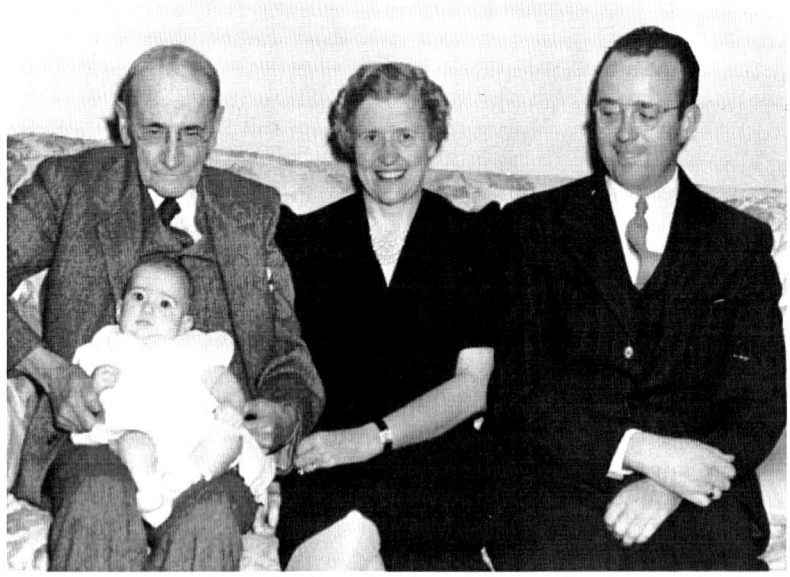

Four generations of the Gardiner family, 1942: Dr. Charles Fox Gardiner, Dorothy Gardiner Hemming, W. D. Hemming Jr. and baby David Hemming. *Photograph from Special Collections, Pikes Peak Library District, courtesy of Mrs. W. D. Hemming.*

Introduction

Notes:

This work is excerpted from *Doctors, Disease and Dying in the Pikes Peak Region* (Colorado Springs: Pikes Peak Library District, 2008).

1. The title phrase, ". . . the trials and tribulations of a hinterland physician of pioneer days. . . ." appears in "Gardiner tells Quill Club of Early-Day Experiences as 'Doctor at Timberline,'" *Colorado Springs Gazette*, January 25, 1939, 6; "Damn it, I wanted to be Ninety," quoted of her father in Dorothy Gardiner Hemming Oral History Interview IV, April 29, 1971, Special Collections, Pikes Peak Library District, Oral History Project, OH-IV Box 2, folder 3; advertisement for *Doctor at Timberline* in *New York Times*, September 8, 1940, 96, William Lyon Phelps, in *Rotarian*. Phelps was a famous literature professor at Yale University, a literary critic, author and preacher. See http://family.phelpsinc.com/bios/william-lyon-phelps.htm.
2. *Colorado Springs Free Press*, August 1, 1947, 1, "Famous Physician and Author Dies; Funeral Saturday."
3. See "Phelps Selects 26 of Best '40 Books," in *New York Times*, August 12, 1940, 13; for "True Picture," see *Colorado Springs Gazette-Telegraph*, November 27, 1938, 10; for Book of the Month Club see *Oakland Tribune*, Oakland, California, October 16, 1938; WorldCat reveals the multiple library locations of Gardiner's book.
4. "Carried Pills to the Hills," "A Book a Day" column by Bruce Catton, *The Clearfield Progress*, Clearfield, Pennsylvania, October 28, 1938.
5. *Colorado Springs Gazette*, January 25, 1939, 6.
6. Ski clubs existed among California's miners from 1861. The first documented competition in Colorado happened in 1883, between miners at the Star Mine in Irwin. In 1886 Crested Butte established a ski club, and held what some consider to be the first American ski meet between Crested Butte and Gunnison ski club racers. See http://www.aspenhistory.org/recre1.html. Snow skiing is the second-largest industry in Colorado, generating over $2 billion annual revenue with eight percent of state employment coming from ski and winter sport. Colorado Ski Country USA, *Economic Impact Study*, March 2004.
7. "Colorado's mining industry directly employs 5,000 persons in the mining industry and generates more than 5,162 jobs in related

industries.... Colorado ranks third among the states in mineral royalty receipts." See http://www.coloradomining.org/COMiningFacts.html.

8. Unpublished manuscript, "Personal History," by Charles Fox Gardiner, n.d.

9. Ibid.

10. Hemming, OH-IV.

11. Austin Flint, Jr. [1836-1915] was a physiologist and educator who in 1861 founded the Bellevue Hospital Medical College where Gardiner earned his M.D. in 1882. Flint served as professor and chair of the Department of Physiology and Microbiology [1861-1897] and was also the surgeon general for the state of New York. See http://www.whonamedit.com/doctor.cfm/2512.html.

12. Billy Edwards [1844–ca. 1908] was one of the most famous lightweight fighters of the mid-nineteenth century, known as "the pugilistic marvel of the age." His image and biography appear on a trading card: Mecca Cigarettes "Champion Athlete & Champion Series;" for nickname "Spider," see Charles Fox Gardiner, "Boxing," CU 36, unpublished manuscript, Special Collections, Pikes Peak Library District; for Featherweight Amateur Boxing Champion, see Jack Schaefer, "Charles Fox Gardiner" in *Heroes Without Glory: Some Goodmen of the Old West* (Boston: Houghton Mifflin Company, 1965), 254.

13. Charles Fox Gardiner, "Canoeing," CU 36.

14. For example, see Sheila M. Rothman, *Living in the Shadow of Death*, 152.

15. Charles Fox Gardiner, "Personal History," CU 36.

16. Charles Fox Gardiner, "Business," CU 36.

17. Hemming, OH-IV, 1; *Colorado Springs Telegraph*, October 12, 1938, 3.

18. Harvey T. Sethman, ed., *A Century of Colorado Medicine 1871–1971* (Denver: Colorado Medical Society, 1971). According to letters from Gardiner's children, Dorothy Gardiner Hemming and Raynor M. Gardiner, Charles Fox Gardiner went to Crested Butte, Colorado, in 1882, remaining there for two years, then moved to Meeker, living there until 1885. However, in a 1901 letter included in the Colorado College Tutt Library Century Chest [transcription 62], Gardiner stated that he "came west in 1883" and to Colorado Springs in 1887.

Introduction

19. The 1883 *Colorado Business Directory* for Crested Butte lists three physicians not including Gardiner; apparently one of the three was an alcoholic.

20. For surgeon for the Colorado Coal and Iron Company, see Schaefer, *Heroes*, 266.

21. Hemming, OH-IV, 2; Aldridge.

22. *Colorado Springs Daily Gazette*, November 22, 1884, 4, announcement of Gardiner–Monteith marriage on November 20, 1884; train timetable; included in a list of Antlers [Hotel] arrivals were Mr. C. F. Gardiner and wife. Gardiner was listed as practicing at Crested Butte in the *1886 Medical and Surgical Directory of the United States* (Detroit: R. L. Polk & Co., 1886). See Patsy R. Page, *Directory of Colorado Physicians, 1886* (Alachua, Florida: Page Publications, 1995).

23. The men's relationship to Gardiner is designated "Batching," rather than "Boarding," which may mean that the men resided at the Gardiner residence but did not take meals there.

24. New York census, 1870, 1880.

25. Schaefer, *Heroes*, 275.

26. Schaefer, ibid.; Hemming, OH-IV, 6.

27. James Monteith appears in the 1885 El Paso County Colorado census, in the 1886 *Colorado Springs City Directory*, suggesting that Daisy's family maintained at least a temporary residence in the city at the northeast corner of Weber and Bijou Streets, and Monteith visited the city in June 1887 (see *Colorado Springs Gazette*, June 19, 1887); James Monteith died in 1890 in New York; from 1892-1896, James Walter Monteith, Daisy's twelve-years-younger brother is listed in the *Colorado Springs City Directory*.

28. *This is What I Remember*, 36.

29. For educational opportunities, see Hemming, OH-IV, 3; Aldridge; *Colorado Springs Gazette*, September 7, 1887, "Dr. Charles F. Gardiner yesterday filed with the county clerk his license to practice medicine and surgery."

30. The 1892 *Colorado Springs City Directory* lists J. W. [James Walter] Monteith, Daisy's younger brother, at 224 East Pikes Peak Avenue, as well as Charles F. Gardiner.

31. *Colorado Springs Gazette*, March 7, 1893; El Paso County Death Register March 3, 1893, states cause of death as consumption lasting for one year.

32. Denise Oldach, *Here Lies Colorado Springs* (Colorado Springs: City of Colorado Springs, Evergreen and Fairview Cemeteries, 1995), 51, 52.

33. Hemming, OH-IV, 3.

34. *Colorado Springs Gazette & Telegraph*, June, 27, 1954, 6, Mrs. C. F. Gardiner obituary; Fanny Anderson Gardiner was born in 1862 in St. Louis and came to Colorado Springs in 1883 with her parents. She was the former Miss Frances Stickney and married Dr. Gardiner in April 1897; *Facts*, Vol. 3, Christmas Edition, 1897, 8.

35. As example, see the excellent biography, *Dr. [Gerald] Webb of Colorado Springs*, by Helen Clapesattle (Boulder: Colorado Associated University Press, 1984).

36. J. Juan Reid, *Colorado College: The First Century, 1874–1974* (Colorado Springs: The Colorado College, *1974*), 47. The college issued annual publications entitled *Colorado College Studies*, containing scientific articles written by its members, 47; Charlie Brown Hershey, *Colorado College 1874–1949* (Colorado Springs: Dentan Printing Company, 1952), Charles Fox Gardiner, Lecturer, 284.

37. "Immunity from Phthisis as Affected by Altitude in Colorado," *American Journal of the Medical Sciences*, 1892, civ, 55; a bibliography of Gardiner's articles appears in *Medical Coloradoana: a Jubilee Volume in Celebration of the Semi-Centennial Anniversary of the Colorado State Medical Society, 1871–1921*, 59.

38. Rothman, 152, quoting Gardiner in "The Sanatory Tent and Its Use in Pulmonary Consumption," *Transactions of the American Climatological Association* 9 (1902): 209; Robert Hoff, *The History of Health Care in the Pikes Peak Region* (Bloomington, Ind.: AuthorHouse, 2005), 32.

39. Clapesattle, 115.

40. Clapesattle, joint statistical study, 366; Colorado Foundation for Research in Tuberculosis, 369.

Charles Fox Gardiner Letter, 1901

CHARLES FOX GARDINER, M. D.
224 PIKE'S PEAK AVENUE,
COLORADO SPRINGS,
OFFICE HOURS { 9.30 TO 10.30 A. M. / 2.30 TO 4.30 P. M. } COLORADO.
TELEPHONE 127.

Saturday Aug 3rd 1901

To my Professional Brothers of the year 2001

Gentlemen

I have been requested to write you a letter and to if possible give you some idea of a doctors life at this place in the present time, as it has been thought the small and insignificant details of our daily life would possibly prove more interesting to you than actual medical history which no doubt you can easily obtain from the mass of data at your disposal —

We live there much as we have during the last fifty years, that is we have to see the sick, and play our social part in the community. The life though of the physician at this place does differ from that of the physician elsewhere because first he has a better climate to be up and shine around in, and second because

Colorado Springs Century Chest Collection, Folder 62, Special Collections, Tutt Library, Colorado College, Colorado Springs, Colorado.

In case any of my descendants are alive and interested in my life —

I am a dutch descendant of Lyon Gardiner (9th?) who came to America 1632 — and who is buried in the town of East Hampton Long Island — I was born in New York City, graduated at Bellevue Hospital Medical College 1882. Served in Charity Hospital — & came west in 1883. Living at first 150 miles from a rail road for several years Among Cow boys and indians then came here. Have two children by my first wife who was Daisy. E. P. M. Gardiner — Raynor Montresor — and Dusty — My second wife Fanny S. Auburn Gardiner. — no children —
I have written a letter, one book Caring the Consumptive being used in several hospitals & in New York — Baltimore — etc.
My father is James Modena — My Grandfather Charles Fox. My G. grandfather Rev. John D.

C. F. Gardiner

Gardiner Letter

Charles Fox Gardiner, M.D.
224 Pike's Peak Avenue
Colorado Springs, Colorado
Office Hours 9:30 to 10:30 A.M
2:30 to 4:30 P.M.
Telephone 127

Saturday Aug 3^d 1901

To my Professional Brothers of the year 2001

Gentlemen

I have been requested to write you a letter and to if possible give you some idea of a doctors life at this place in the present time, as it has been thought the small and insignificant details of our daily life would possibly prove more interesting to you than actual medical history which no doubt you can easily obtain from the mass of data at your disposal—

We live then much as we have during the last fifty years, that is we have to see the sick, and play our social part in the community. The life though of the physician at this place does differ from that of the physician elsewhere because first he has a better climate to be out and drive around in, and second because the people he treats have as a rule one disease more than any other, pulmonary tuberculosis, and from this fact we have many of us, become specialists in healing this disease of the lungs. Our patients come from all over the world to be cured in our dry air and sunshine, this is a cure in a large percent of cases of consumption during the first stage of the disease, and in fact today we rely in all countries on plenty of food and fresh air as a cure, we unfortunately have no other agent of anything like equal value—I have enclosed a chart showing number of days a pulmonary invalid can be out doors, and also a diet list I give my patients, which is taken from my book "Care of the Consumptive, 1900."

My day is spent briefly as follows, after a breakfast at 8.30 I read & write and see patients at my office which is in my house until 10.30 a.m. Our charges are for an office visit $2.00 visit to house $3.00. An examinations of chest first time $10.00 a second examination 5.00. I then drive about town seeing my patients, as the town is built largely with lawns about the houses and the environment decidedly rural and country like, and as many of the people I treat are cultivated & refined, the task I have in my daily work is neither arduous nor disagreeable as a rule—although many of the cases I see are hopelessly ill with consumption and for that reason my sympathies are strongly drawn upon, but even then, they are as a rule bright and full of hope—

The physicians drive a horse and buggie as a rule, a few use motor carriages, but electric are not practical here yet, and steam freezes up in cold weather, while gasoline make a noise and unpleasant smell, a few (one or two) occasionally ride horseback and I did regularly for a number of years when I first came here in 1887 but I drive a two-wheeled top gig with one or two horses, and as the present town is not over 2½ miles in any one direction I seldom have far to go—

I drop in at the El Paso Club & see the men often for a half hour or so, and then back to lunch at one or half after at my house then patients call until 4 o'clock when I drive again to see people or often take my wife for a drive in the country as far as Broadmoor or the canons—The evenings are spent at home or dining with friends, generally I study from 10 to 12, and our El Paso Co. Medical Society meets once a month when papers are read and discussed. At [least?] once a year I go to N.Y. City where I was born in 1857 the trip taking three days and nights and generally attend some medical convention to talk & see the best men and so keep up with the times—This life in Colorado Springs from a medical mans standpoint is not burdened with the rush and anxiety of a medical mans life in a large city like Philadelphia or New York (now called Manhattan) but it has a dash of country & fresh air, and a [leisure?] to enjoy Gods beautiful scenery all about, which to my mind gives it a charm and advantage all its own—

I hope the future will bring a sanitary science that will render most diseases harmless—and when you smile at our work and

Gardiner Letter

no doubt wonder how we could have been so blind as not to see and know all you do, remember when you smile that we did our best as you are doing. And so gentlemen God bless & keep you one and all, and "we who are about to die salute you," who are not yet born —

With best wishes & kind regards for you in the year 2001

Sincerely yours

Charles Fox Gardiner

In case any of my descendents are alive and interested in my life —

I am a direct descendent of Lyon Gardiner (9th) who came to America 1632 — and who is buried in the town of East Hampton Long Island — I was born in New York City, graduated at Bellevue Hospital Medical College 1882. Served in Charity Hospital — came west in 1883. Living at first 150 miles from a rail road for several years among cowboys and indians then came here, Have two children by my first wife who was Daisy E. P. M. Gardiner — Raynor Monteith — and Dorothy — My second wife Fanny S. Anderson Gardiner. — No children —

I have written a little: one book, Care of the Consumptive being used in several hospitals etc. in New York — Baltimore — etc.

My father is James Madison — my grandfather Charles Fox. My g.grandfather Rev. John D.

C. F. Gardiner

Doctor at Timberline

Preface

It is now some fifty years since I started as a young physician to practice among the silver mines of western Colorado, in the heart of the Rocky Mountains. I lived at a high altitude, often above timber line, with deep snow covering the ground for nine months of the year. The pioneer miners lived a life of hardship, and bravely faced dangers that, seen through the eyes of a medical man who lived among them as I did, may have some historical interest.

After practicing in the silver camps I moved to the cattle country at a lower altitude of about six thousand feet. There I practiced among the cowboys on the open range, in a wild unsettled region one hundred fifty miles from the nearest railroad. I made my home in a small town still called a "cow town," and made my professional calls on horseback. By living with these people as I did, rather than as an infrequent visitor to hunt or fish for a few weeks and then return to civilization again, I had an opportunity to study the men and women who did the actual wilderness breaking for the settlers who came after them. Among them were all classes, from the college professor to the common cowpuncher. There were Indians, hunters, outlaws, gamblers; men who were fleeing the law; men who would shoot you as they would a rabbit; men rough in speech and action, unlettered, uncouth, and yet with as fine a regard for honor, honesty, and truth as the finest gentlemen in the land. With these I ate and slept; I suffered with them on long rides through heat, cold, and dangers of flood and fire; I mended their bodies, and so touched their souls.

I was the only doctor for over a hundred miles around; and some of my long rides through what was then a wilderness may be worth writing about, as they throw some light on the life of the old-time cowpuncher and the work of the pioneer physician, both now faded into a picture of fables far from the truth. I am told that in writing of my experiences I must at least mention who I am and why I deliberately selected such wild and uncomfortable surroundings in which to practice medicine.

I was born in New York City from an old, well-known New England family dating from 1632—an only child, delicate, sensitive, always reading books, and, no doubt, spoiled and ill fitted for any rough struggle in the world. I was always thin and delicate-looking. I never have weighed more than one hundred ten pounds with my clothes on, although I am five feet seven inches tall; my father was just the same, and my mother weighed but one hundred pounds, so I was naturally of light weight.

At about sixteen I suddenly made up my mind that if I could not be big and robust, at least I could, by constant practice, become wiry and tireless. This, no doubt, was the result of some inferiority complex. At any rate, I stuck to the idea. For nine years I put my slim body through a course of violent exercise, and it is a wonder I did not injure myself. I went to Wood's Gymnasium in Twenty-eighth Street, and put in two hours a day. In those days this was a favorite resort for business and professional men who needed exercise to keep fit, and some of the leading men in the city, both socially and financially, used to come to the gymnasium from four to six o'clock every afternoon and run on the track, work on the parallel bars, and use the generous supply of all kinds of apparatus. My father had been present on the opening night in 1858, so I was always welcomed, and knew Mr. Woods, the owner, very well. The famous Austin Flint had a class he directed and led on the parallel bars, and this noted physiologist was very kind and helpful to me in my efforts to train my muscles. I remember his remark to me, "You can never increase your size by exercise, but you can make your body as tough as a whipcord."

Some of the stars of Barnum's circus used the gymnasium in the mornings to perfect themselves in their feats of tumbling

Preface

and trapeze work. They took a liking to me and very kindly taught me to do forward and back somersaults and horizontal bar work. I also took lessons in boxing for five years from Billy Edwards, the noted prize fighter, and in summer I went alone on long walking trips in the Catskill and White Mountains. I also took up long-distance running, and gradually, by years of practice, hardened my thin, frail body so that, although I was not big and strong, I was very active and could tire out many of my stronger friends. I always had a great desire to be an explorer. I read all the books I could find on the subject, and men who went to the unknown parts of the earth were my heroes. In a way, I was preparing my body to stand the exposure and fatigue of such a life, and when I took my long walking trips I slept in one blanket, made a fire in the rain, learned to use an axe and a rifle, and studied how to care for myself.

I studied medicine and was graduated from Bellevue Medical College. I was an interne in Charity Hospital, and then a surgeon at the prison on Blackwells Island. I also was for six months in the outdoor surgical service in New York Hospital.

I was always determined to go to some wild place, far from cities, and at last started for Colorado with very little money, no experience; and to the mingled amusement and disquiet of my friends, I intended to try it for a year or so. I have stayed fifty years! I do not regret it for an instant. I have had the delight of seeing great snow-covered mountains, of breathing pure air, of having the sunshine and blue sky greet me day after day, and of knowing men in the rough—simple and true and unafraid.

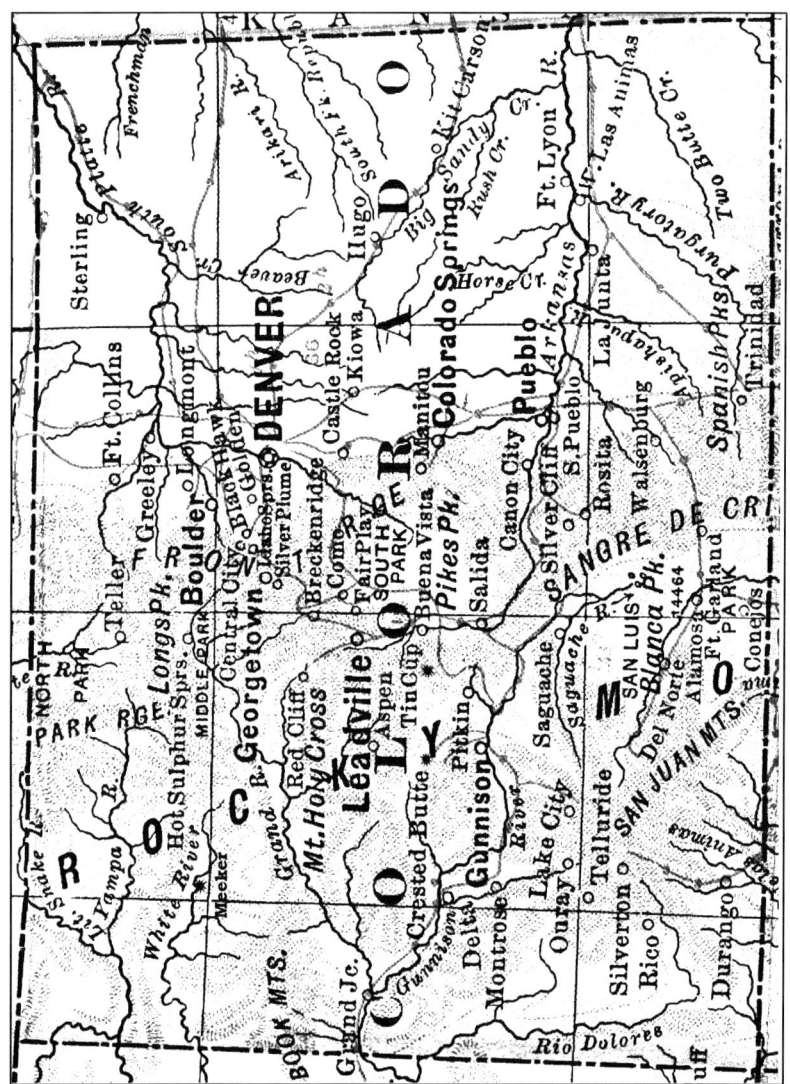

Map of Colorado from *Barnes' Complete Geography* published in 1885 by James Monteith, "author of geographies, atlases, maps, wall-maps, *Easy Lessons in Popular Science* and *Popular Science Reader*." James Monteith was the father of Emma "Daisy" Palmer Monteith. Charles Fox Gardiner married Daisy at Grace Episcopal Church in Colorado Springs on November 20, 1884. This map shows the location of Crested Butte, where Charles Gardiner lived in 1883, and the town of Meeker, where Daisy and Charles settled and started their family.

Chapter 1

A Tenderfoot Doctor on Ski and Bronco

One January day I stood, shivering with cold, at an altitude of ten thousand feet above sea level, and looked at the strange collection of log cabins, rough lumber stores, saloons, and buildings with false fronts, that were built on each side of a main street. The town was in a little valley. On all sides the big snow mountains shut it in. Massive snow slopes and rocky summits towering above seemed about to fall and crush it. The plank sidewalks were built along the street and were raised some two feet above the ground, like walks I had seen in seaside resorts. This was done in order that the snow might be shoveled into the street more easily. The fall of snow up in these regions was so heavy during about eight or nine months of the year that it was necessary to shovel it off the roofs of all buildings or it would crush them. Then the snow was shoveled into the street, so that in the middle of winter the street consisted of a mound of snow fifteen feet high extending its entire length, shutting off all view across the street, save where openings had been cut. In fact, the street could be used for wagons in summer only, when the snow had melted. This depth of snow was a constant wonder to me. Some sections of the mountains were worse than others, but on the western slopes at an elevation of eight thousand feet or more, many of the camps were snowbound all winter. The snow, when I arrived, was six feet deep on the level ground, and drifts covering the telegraph poles were not unusual.

The question of altitude in the Rocky Mountains made a vast difference in the cold and the snowfall during the winter. The higher you go in the mountains, the colder it will be, and the deeper the snowfall. This is much more marked on the western slope of the Rocky Mountains in Colorado, where the winds from the Pacific carrying moisture-laden clouds are arrested by the high mountains and their moisture is precipitated in the form of snow.

Where I lived, among the peaks of the Elkhorn Range, this feature was very marked and the snowfall unusually heavy. Deep snow made it impossible to clear the roads or trails and, very early in the history of these camps, the long, narrow snowshoe, the Norwegian ski, was introduced. Nothing surprised me more in my first sight of this strange settlement than to see people going about on skis. Everyone used them, quite as a matter of course, and slid over the top of the deep snow with the utmost skill. Even little children just able to walk were flying about on their little snowshoes and playing games in the most natural way in the world. It was amusing to see them fall off and sink almost out of sight in the soft snow and be pulled out again on their skis by laughing playmates. When not in use, these skis were stuck upright in any snowbank where, like a thin line of bare trees, they swayed in the wind.

Looking at all the strange sights, I grew chilled in my New York clothes. The sun was bright, the sky was very blue, but the temperature was down to zero, so I asked the way to the hotel. I was shown a large, square, unpainted structure with the usual ugly false front. Painted on it was a sign, "Mountain Hotel."

As I picked up my bag and walked along the boardwalk I could hear the boards under my feet creaking from the cold. I had gone only a little way when, walking rather rapidly to keep warm,

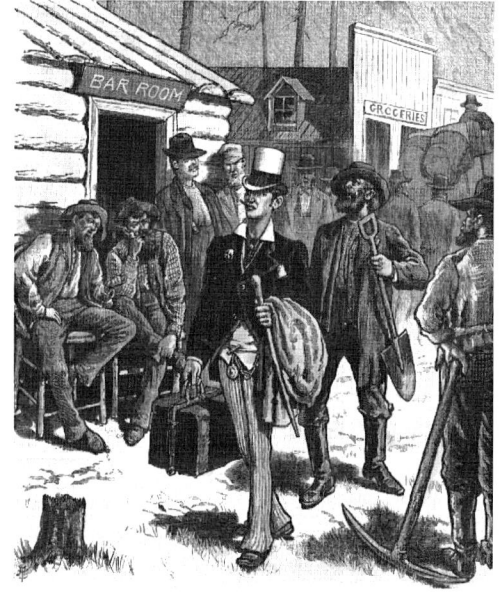

I suddenly felt as if I had been running a mile. I could not get my breath! Gasping, I sat down on my bag and unbuttoned my coat, feeling faint. Then I realized that it was the thin air at ten thousand feet acting on my lungs, which were used to sea level. I saw people smile as they passed by. I suppose I looked very much a tenderfoot as I sat there panting for breath, my dark overcoat, derby hat, and polished shoes in marked contrast to the flannel shirts and big boots of the people I saw. Their faces were burnt red with the sun, and their every action showed their health and strength. A miner came striding along the walk, his skis on one shoulder, on his way to some mine far up amid the snow peaks. On his back he carried his pack—a large gunny sack filled with provisions—and on this I saw a box with a printed notice, "Giant Powder No. 3. Danger!" A nice load of destruction to carry over slippery mountain trails!

As I was passing by a saloon, a man opened the door to come out on the walk, and with him came a fog of tobacco smoke, whisky fumes, and steam from wet clothes. I caught a glimpse of the interior. I saw a big bar at one end; the barkeeper in a red shirt, his arms bare, mixing drinks; a sanded floor; and men sitting around little tables playing poker. There was a confused murmur of voices, the clatter of poker chips thrown on tables, the scraping of heavy boots on the floor, and the door closed again. I was a bit shocked at this gambling going on in broad daylight, open to anyone. I certainly was green and innocent about the West at first!

The street was very quiet. There were no wagons, no horses; only footsteps on the board sidewalks, or the bark of a dog. I heard a distant rumble that sounded like thunder in the mountains; it grew heavier, the walk under my feet shook, and then, with a last roar, the sound stopped. I wondered if it could be an earthquake; no one on the walk seemed to notice it so I asked a passing miner what that noise was.

"Why, man alive," he exclaimed, "don't you know snowslides when you hear them?"

So for the first time I heard that growl of the mountain giant that strikes terror to those who are in its path as, with a roar like heavy artillery, tons and tons of snow start sliding down the steep slopes far up above timber line and, gathering speed and weight in the rush, go like an express train, breaking through heavy trees as if they were straws, and at last, pile up with a crash in the bottom of some gulch, a mass of dirty snow and broken trees one hundred feet high, groaning and cracking as if in pain, until at last it sinks to a frozen silence.

I reached the hotel at last. There was a long porch across the front, and arrivals were stamping their feet and sticking their snowshoes in the snow in front. I could not see inside, for the windows were thickly covered with frost. I opened the front door and entered a big hall that served as office and general lounging place. At one side there was a counter with a book to register in, and a key rack on the wall. In the middle was a big, red-hot stove, and around it a group of men were seated in plain kitchen chairs, tilted back, their boots on the rail of the stove, steaming in the heat. All were talking loudly about some new mine just discovered. I walked over to the desk, where I saw a man who looked like the proprietor. He smiled very kindly as he pushed the book up for me to sign. When he saw that I was a doctor from New York he grew very friendly. He told me that he was from Montreal, Canada, and had run this hotel for a year as a venture. His name was Ben McLoid. He was a nice-looking man of fifty, with small, rather delicate face and figure. Evidently he was well educated. With a smile he remarked that no doubt I found everything very rough at first, as he had, but that I would grow to like it. As he evidently considered me a young doctor of some means who was traveling in the West for a change from city life, I grew more and more uncomfortable.

I could not bear to sail under false colors, and as I had but little money in my pocket, I determined to make a clean breast of it to this friendly landlord. Leaning over the counter and speaking in a low voice so as not to be overheard by the crowd around the stove, I told my friend that all I had in the world was fifteen dollars. After that was gone I had to make my living, and, handing the money to him, I asked him to keep me at his hotel as long as it lasted. The effect of this confession on my host

McLoid was immediate and startling. He looked at me and then at the money I had given him. At first he was astonished. Then he burst out laughing, calling out to the men around the stove, "Say, boys, come up here; I have a good one to tell you."

At once the crowd came over in a body, laughing as they surrounded me, and asking McLoid "what the hell was up." I was both angry and embarrassed at being made fun of, and was about to tell McLoid what I thought about him when, in a hurried whisper, he said, "Wait a minute, Doctor. Please wait."

"Gentlemen," said McLoid, addressing the men, "this is a doctor from New York. In place of running a bluff on me with his good clothes, he hands me fifteen dollars, says it is all he has, and wants to board it out as far as it will go. Now, boys, I never had such a straight story told me before, and I want to tell him he can stay here all winter, and damn his fifteen dollars!" How that crowd laughed! They crowded me into the bar in a back room, and I had a drink with them, all joking and friendly.

At supper, which was served at a long table in the dining room, and was announced by the ringing of a big bell in the hall, I noticed a strange bit of etiquette observed by these miners at table. They had first wet and brushed their hair down slick. As the bell rang they hurriedly seated themselves at the table and devoured the food in such a hurry you would think they had not a moment to lose. The silence was profound. Apparently it was bad form to speak at meals. I made a few feeble efforts to converse with my next neighbors, but this created such notice—not to say disapproval—among the other guests, that I soon followed the custom and was as silent as the rest.

After supper we all gathered around the stove again. My trunk having been carried to my room, I mentioned that I was going to unpack my things. Several of the men got up with me, saying in the most natural way, "All right, Doc, we're coming to see what you have in that trunk." It was so simple and childlike that I could not object, and their enjoyment as I unpacked and spread my belongings around was too evident to spoil. Some of my clothes were the cause of much joking. My instruments were handled with serious interest. But the climax came when, from the bottom of my trunk, I hauled forth an old suit of oilskins I had used in fishing off Long Island the summer before. Now, my audience happened to be men who had never been near salt water in their lives, and when I showed them the suit—trousers and coat, with a sou'wester to match, several sizes too big for me—all a bright, shining yellow with a stamp on each garment in black letters, "Fish Brand," these inland boys went wild. Nothing would do but each in turn must put on the suit and parade up and down the room to the delight of the others. At last the party broke up, and they all clumped downstairs making an awful noise, calling out what fun they had had, and "Good night, Doc."

As I turned in to sleep on the cold, lumpy bed, I thought what boys these Rocky Mountain miners were, after all, and I felt that I was going to like the West. Just as I was going to sleep there was a deep rumble from the mountains that rattled the windowpanes in my room, and I knew that a snowslide was roaring its mighty way down some big mountain.

I was awakened in the morning by revolver shots in front of the hotel. I could hear shouts and yelling and men running on the boardwalk. I felt sure there was a gun battle going on, so I ran to the window and scraped a hole in the frost that covered the glass. But my room was at the back of the hotel, and I could see nothing. Trembling with excitement and cold, I threw on my clothes, grabbed my first-aid bag, and ran downstairs prepared for battle, murder, and sudden death. The main hall was empty and, running out onto the front porch, I found it crowded with men, all laughing at something going on in the street. I pushed my way to the front, and there I stood, too astonished to move. Some wag among the company at my rooms the night before had stolen my precious oilskin suit as he had left and had, with much skill, stuffed the suit with old papers and rags so that it looked like a bloated man. He had then suspended this weird figure by a rope over a telegraph wire about twenty feet up in the air, right over the middle of the main street. There it swayed back and forth in the wind, a striking imitation of a man who had been hanged. A large placard had been fastened to the back, and in big black letters was printed, "High water doc."

Men had scrambled on top of the mound of snow that filled the street and were shooting their revolvers at the swaying figure. Every bullet that hit the figure made a big hole and tore out some of the rags or paper with which it was filled, and at every successful shot roars of approval went up from the crowd. I was seen at once as I appeared in front of the hotel. Laughter and yells greeted me as I stood in open-mouthed wonder at the strange scene and saw my oilskin suit torn to tatters. Of course I could see that it was all fun—part of the horseplay so dear to rough, outdoor men like these miners—and I also realized that I must meet it in the same spirit or lose caste with them for all time. So I shouted out, "The drinks are on me, boys! Come inside," and led the joyful band to the bar where my fifteen dollars was soon poured down thirsty throats amid general good nature and many a "Here's to you, Doc." So the affair went off very well, after all. I was rapidly being educated to the standards of the Western mining camps.

After a few weeks in my new surroundings I found that making a living by practicing in a mining town was not so easy as I had hoped. There were two other doctors practicing in camp and, although they were rather rough specimens, they were ahead of me, were much older men, and did practically all there was to do. I knew that their knowledge of up-to-date medicine was sadly lacking, and that mining occupied most of their time, but they had a knowledge of human nature and a business sense that gave success, so I was left out in the cold. I was also finding out to my sorrow that there were diseases in the West I had never heard of or seen in the New York hospitals.

One day a young miner, just arrived from South Carolina, was brought to me, very ill with a fever. He vomited, had chills, had a temperature of $103\frac{1}{2}$ degrees, and that night, became delirious, growing worse every hour. Athough I examined him with every method I knew, his symptoms were so unusual and confusing that I was utterly at a loss to give his disease a name. Naturally I hated to admit it, being very young and dreading to let people see that I was unable to make a diagnosis. Tired out and discouraged, my confidence at its lowest ebb, I was sitting by my patient, who was raving and trying to get out of bed. At this stage of the game, in walked Uncle Billy, whose real name was William Webster McConnell, but known to everyone as "Uncle Billy."

Uncle Billy was one of those unique characters that have now passed into history. I had been of some little service to him at our first meeting, and he was more than grateful. He had come around to see if he could help with my patient and, as he stood regarding that poor youth struggling on the bed, he turned to me with a smile on his lined old face and said, "Doc, I bet you don't know what ails the feller, do you?"

I believe I blushed, but I had the grace to say, "No, I don't."

Uncle Billy was amused, but too kind to show it. "Why, Doc," he said, "that boy is a 'Tarheel' from Carolina, and he's got the cow sickness; some of my kinfolks was took with it when I was a kid, and a right smart number died of it."

Fortunately my patient recovered, because of my nursing, rather than as the result of any medical skill for, apparently, drugs did not have much effect. Since then this cow sickness—such a mystery to me, for I could find no reference to it in medical literature—has been carefully and scientifically studied and is now known to be a severe infection from cows or their milk. Now, as then, the favored treatment is good nursing. Uncle Billy saved the day for me that time, and we became good friends.

Uncle Billy was a bachelor of sixty years or more, tall and straight, with a loose-jointed, angular frame. Born in Tennessee, he had fought in the Civil War for the South, and then had roamed all over the West. He had been shot a number of times, had been among cattlemen and Indians, and had at last come to a comparatively peaceful life in our camp, doing a little mining and running a store called a drugstore, where he slept and cooked his meals. He wore his hair long, had a big gray mustache and goatee, and dressed in an old Prince Albert frock coat. The latter was much worn and faded, but evidently he fondly thought it was in style. It made him feel quite civilized, although his big cowboy hat and his knee boots detracted a little from this ideal.

I often wondered what my New York friends would think of this friend of mine. I must confess that he was very dirty, that his habits were rather free and easy, that he chewed tobacco and spat anywhere, and that his daily consumption of raw whisky was enough to kill outright any average healthy man. But this was all on the surface; the real man was another person, often to be seen only in his smile and the kindly look in his eyes. He was one of those pure and simple souls who told the truth by instinct, would give the coat off his back to help a friend, and thought every woman and child pure, beautiful, and an object of worship. In addition to this, he had a curious intuition regarding human ills. Whether it was born in him or acquired by his intense sympathy with suffering I could never determine. But one thing was sure: in spite of his ignorance of all medical knowledge he could, by a sort of sixth sense, read a sick person like a book. With wounds, his concoctions made by boiling certain roots in water and applying the infusion were certainly remarkable. He would never tell me what he used, and he never charged a penny for their use. I believe he got his remedies from the Indians with whom he had, at one time, lived for several years. At any rate, I used them and was not ashamed to confess that they were far more efficacious than anything I had. As he saved my life later in the year when I had blood poisoning, I feel rather positive on the subject.

Then I came up against another new disease—new, at least, to me. The miners traveling over the vast white snow fields, which glittered with a cruel light in the sunshine of high altitudes, were often attacked. Showing first by a redness of the lids and a profuse flow of tears, the disease rapidly developed into a fearful, stabbing pain in the eyeballs, loss of sight; and in severe cases the patient became crazy for a time, running about and dashing into everything in his way. The first case I had was a powerful, sandy-haired young Swede, who was led along on snowshoes and supported by two companions. I thought he had been powder burnt, but when I tried to lift his eyelids apart to see his eyes, he gave a scream as the light caught his eyes, flung himself on the ground, and acted like a man in convulsions. His comrades told me the trouble they had had with him, and I had him put in a dark room. There was no cocaine in those days—only a solution of sulphate of zinc to put in the eyes—but he recovered, and I had seen a disease new to me—snow blindness.

The next three months I did not have any practice. I was in debt, and things seemed to be going rather badly with me. I passed the time by learning how to walk on snowshoes. In fact, when snow covers the whole country around you to a depth of six feet, with drifts in places so deep that the telegraph poles are buried, the only way to get about at all is to use snowshoes. And even then there is always danger of breaking a snowshoe. If this happened on a trip over a wild section of the country where deep snow stretched for miles in every direction, and above timber line where there was no wood for a fire, and the night temperature below zero, you had to mend that broken snowshoe or perish. Most old-timers carried some rivets, or screws, and a gimlet to mend a broken shoe. But I have known several cases of men who could not mend a shoe, who, after trying for hours to break a trail through the snow, became exhausted and froze to death. A long furrow like a ditch leading up to their bodies was mute evidence of their pathetic struggles in this cruel and soft blanket, as gradually and silently it dragged them down and covered their last feeble struggles like a white pall.

The web shoe is used in Canada, but in the high altitudes in the Rocky Mountains, on the western side of the Great Divide, where I lived, I never saw anything used but the long Norwegian shoes, or what are known as "skis." They were about seven or eight feet long by five or six inches wide, and curved up at the end. They are the only practical snowshoes to use in a big open country where there is very little timber, bushes, or undergrowth to go through. There were often long, sloping mountains to go over, where for miles you could coast along on skis without effort and at a speed that was much faster than was possible with web shoes. Of course, going up these long hills was another matter; what we did was to make long zigzags like a railroad. For a brake we fastened a piece of deerskin on the under side of the shoes, with the hair pointing back. If the shoes slipped back on a steep climb, the hair would be turned the wrong way and stick out so as to hold the shoe.

We did not use the two canelike sticks with disks at the end, such as are used now. We all used an ash pole about six to seven feet long, and when going down a steep place we rode this pole as would a boy, playing horse. This acted as a brake. When going on the level we used this pole on one side as in poling a boat through the water. This use of the pole was not only a help, but also aided in keeping one's balance. I believe that the Norwegian miners who came to the mountains first introduced the skis in the mining section of Colorado. I do know that they were in common use in 1879, and made possible the working of mines in winter, for by their use food could be packed in to snowbound camps. They made it possible for one to go from camp to camp, across mountains and snow fields impossible to travel over for six to seven months of the year.

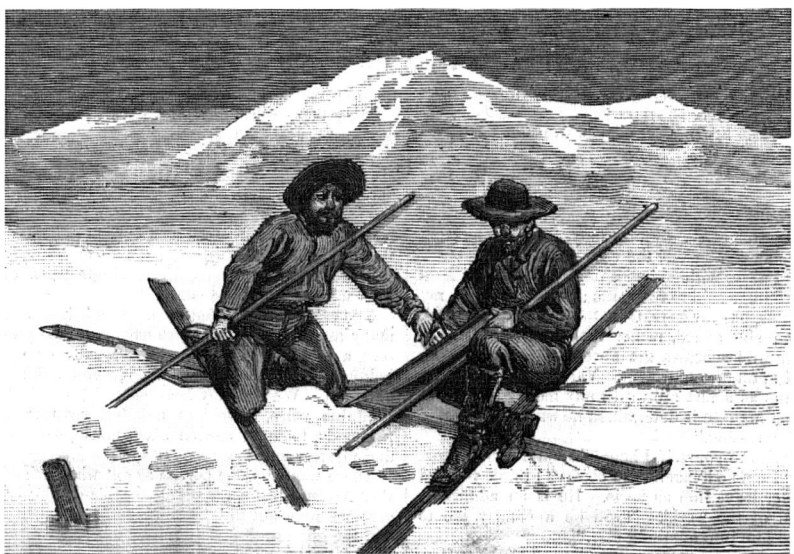

We had no trouble in buying skis. Several Norwegians, who had made a business of making skis in Norway, established their shops in camp and turned out the best skis I have ever seen. They were made of clear-grained ash, straight as an arrow, with just enough spring. They were very strong; their lines and curves were so nicely adjusted that they were works of art. Each pair of skis was made to order. The size of your feet, your height and weight, and, more than all, how you were to use them, were all carefully considered. A miner who would use his shoes when packing heavy weights had skis of different make from a man who would travel light, or who would use his skis only for races or sport. Some skis had a single groove running along the underside to prevent sideslips—never more than one groove, and the expert would not have that. The sliding surface was rubbed down as smooth as silk, and then wax was applied by a hot iron and polished until it shone like a mirror.

I was much interested in the snowshoeing. I had never seen or heard of skis in the East at that time, and I took to the sport because I liked it, and because it was absolutely necessary for me to learn if I had to go on a call to some other camp. I had a hard time at first. There was a mountain just back of the town—a big, round mountain that rose up one thousand feet and provided a steep slide down to the valley. About half the people in town would shut up shop early in the afternoon and take their skis to this mountain. It was a long, hard climb to the top. From there, as you looked down at the valley and town so far below, the people looked like ants moving about. The edge of the mountain at your feet was so steep that it seemed as if you were looking straight down a precipice into space. On your shoes and going down, the speed was so terrific and the wind against you so strong that you felt exactly as if you were falling from some high cliff. At the bottom you glided on a big, almost-level plane clear across the valley for two miles or so. The best time was in the late winter, when a thick crust that would hold up a man formed on the surface of the snow, with just enough snow on top to make the shoes hold. The way small boys would give a yell, plunge down the long slide with the utmost ease and skill, managing their little skis like veterans, would make me, in my novice days, green with envy. It was a fearful moment when, taking my courage in both hands, I slipped over this edge and went flying down so rapidly it took my breath away, the snow plumes rising from the front of my shoes in long ribbons. The valley seemed to rush up to meet me, and it was no time at all before I was gliding over a level field, safe and very proud of myself.

In these days of ski running and jumping on prepared slides, it would seem that I am making quite a fuss about coming down a mountain, but I fancy some of these ski runners would have treated this mountain slide with considerable respect if they could have taken it in the old days. We descended a slope one thousand feet high at an angle of forty-five degrees, and the speed was about as fast as one could go and stay on the shoes. No pole was used on this run, and often one run was enough, for it took so long to climb up. I had one bad fall when a dog got in the way, which tossed me some twenty feet. I broke through the crust into the soft snow, so was not hurt. It was like falling into a feather bed, but my right knee was twisted as my shoe slued around crossways to the trail. I was laid up for a week.

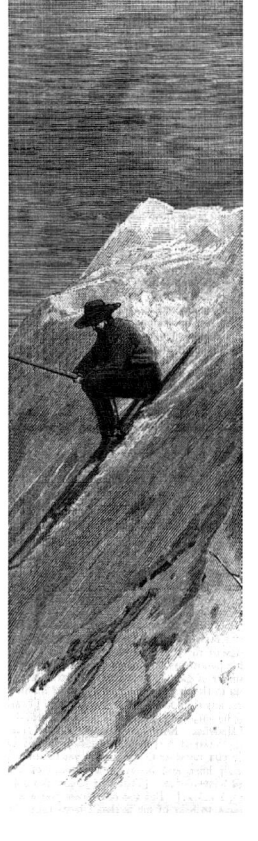

Then we sent to Montreal for six toboggans. When they came we had some glorious sliding, to the amazement of the old-timers, who had never seen such things before, and refused point-blank to risk their lives on them. So the long winter passed, and I enjoyed the freedom and new experiences, but was worried over not being able to establish a paying practice.

At last the cloud lifted a little, and in a way I never imagined. Mr. Collins, a mining engineer who owned a big interest in some of the paying mines over in the Bald Mountain district, came into camp one day suffering from toothache. Mr. Collins was a man of thirty-five, from Boston, who appeared and acted like a gentleman. He said he could not spare the time to go to Denver to see a dentist. He did not want to lose the tooth, and he asked if I could do anything to tide him over and stop the pain without sacrificing it. He declared he would gladly give a hundred dollars for relief. Now, a hundred dollars looked as big as a wagon wheel to me just then, and I got busy in my new role as dentist. I found the hole in his aching molar and put in some pure carbolic acid. The pain stopped. It was an old trick that I had learned from the dentist at the prison in New York. Mr. Collins was delighted, had a good sleep, and went off happy, with some of the acid to use himself, telling me he would come back in a week, as I had requested. I knew the relief would be only temporary, for the pulp, or nerve, was exposed. I sent to Denver for some soft dental filling, and on his return I filled the hole in his tooth, and hoped it would stay for a month anyway. I was lucky, and Mr. Collins paid me the hundred dollars. He also told some others, with the result that I filled teeth and got together a little money.

 I built a small board office on the main street, put out a sign with gold letters on a blue-sky background—a most awful creation—that swung over my front door and across the boardwalk on a long iron support. I was glad none of my doctor friends in New York could see it, but I was only conforming to the custom of the country. All the other doctors had very much the same signs; mine was painted by a stranded Frenchman out of gratitude for my pulling him through a severe attack of delirium tremens. I built a bunk against the wall on one side of the little room at the back, where I slept, and this side of my little house was built only a foot or so from a saloon next door. Both buildings were of rough boards, about one inch thick. Every night as I tried to sleep in my bunk, I could hear the shouts of the men in the saloon, the pounding of their big boots on the floor, the rattle of counters, and the general sounds of a rough crowd making a night of it. Often this kept up until daylight; the buildings were so thin that the sound came through to me as if I were in the saloon. This place had a bad reputation and was

A Tenderfoot Doctor

known as the Slaughter Pen because of the number of men who had been shot and killed while drinking and gambling there.

One night I was at the hotel rather late and, hearing cries and people running, I went out and found a crowd collected in front of the Slaughter Pen. There had been a row over the cards, and some wild shooting. One man had been shot in the arm. The other doctors were inside attending to the wounded man, so I went into my house and undressed. When I started to get into my bunk, I was surprised and alarmed to find my blankets with several bullet holes in them, and my bunk covered with splinters of wood.

During the shooting that had occurred next door in my absence several bullets had gone through the side of the saloon and my wall, tearing big holes in the planks and passing through my blankets, scattering wood splinters all about my room. If I had been in my bunk during this shooting I would have been

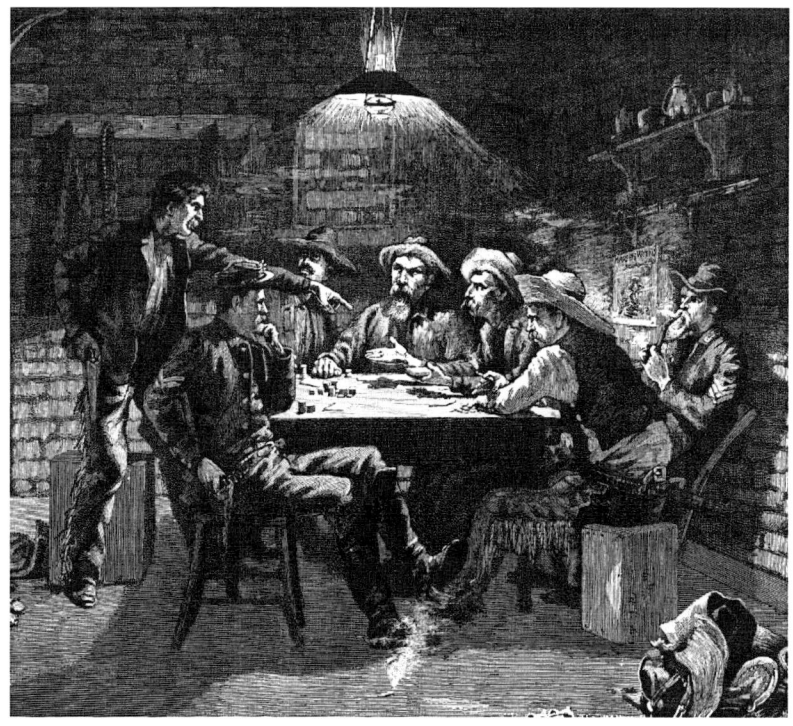

shot or badly wounded. Early the next morning I got to work and built a sort of bulletproof screen of boards, with sand rammed down between it and my side wall, so that I would be safe in the future when the crowd got to shooting in the saloon. Of course the boys had a lot of fun over this "fort" of mine, as they called it, but I never bothered about their jokes, and could turn in and sleep without fear of being shot by mistake some night.

I was having rather a hard struggle to make a living, and my financial resources were coming to an end when luck again turned up something in my favor. It was, as usual, in a way I had never dreamed of. My first venture not strictly in the line of my profession was dentistry. Now, of all things, I was summoned to doctor a cow! I was rapidly learning to take what fate ordered and not to be surprised at anything that occurred in a Western mining camp.

One thing early remarked in these towns was the absence of horses and cows during the period of heavy snowfall. Early in the autumn all horses and cattle were driven out from the high camps to lower and warmer valleys where the snowfall was light and where grazing was possible all winter long. Arriving in the dead of winter as I had, I was surprised to see how quiet the country seemed with no riding or driving, only the soft swish of snowshoes as people passed over the deep mantle that covered the ground. I was certain that not a horse or a cow had been in the town for months, so imagine my surprise to find that one cow had been living within a hundred yards of my own place!

Tom Baxter, owner of the Little Annie, a silver mine on Baldy Mountain, was a keen miner, formerly of New York City. He now lived with his wife and baby a short distance from me. They were pleasant people, fond of reading, and I often dropped in for a visit. One morning Mrs. Baxter called me in to see her baby, who had some stomach upset, as babies will, and of course I asked her what she was feeding the baby. To my surprise, she said, "Milk," and, never dreaming of fresh milk, I was holding forth on the evils of condensed milk when she said, "Why, Doctor, we have our own cow. My husband kept her in camp this winter because I made such a fuss over the baby's having fresh milk."

"How on earth do you keep her?" I asked. "I have never seen a sign of a cow all winter."

"Well, we have, Doctor, and if you care to, Tom will show you the cow." So when Tom came in his wife told him, and Tom laughed.

"Come along, Doctor, and I will show you the mystery." So off we went on our snowshoes about two hundred yards out from the town. I had begun to think that Tom was having a joke on me, for there was nothing in sight but the long, unbroken expanse of white snow as level as a billiard table all around us. Tom, with a smile at my puzzled look, said, "Doctor, do you see that hole in the snow? Well, my cow is down that hole." Then I noticed a hole about two feet wide not far off. When we reached it I saw that a ladder led down a place very much like a mining shaft, and when we stuck our snowshoes in the snow and went down the ladder, the mystery was clear to me. Tom had built a stable of logs covered with a flat dirt roof for his cow in the summer. The stable was low—only about high enough to stand up in—and during the winter the falling snow had gradually grown so deep that it had covered the stable and was a foot deep on the roof. Looking over the snow field you could not see any stable at all.

After the snow covered the roof, Tom got tired of digging a deep hole to reach the door, and just cut a sort of trap door in the middle of the roof, put a ladder down, and got to his cow that way. He carried water down to the cow twice a day, and had one end of the stable filled with baled hay to feed her. He milked her and carried the milk home, first up the ladder and then on snowshoes. The little stable was quite comfortable. Tom said it never grew cold enough to freeze inside, even if it were twenty below zero outside, for the deep snow all over it made a perfect protection, and the warm body of the cow kept the temperature at about fifty degrees, while the hole in the roof gave enough light and air. Although it was only a stable, it seemed quite cozy and homelike to me. No wind could get in, and it put me in mind of the snowhouses the Eskimos build in the Far North. I thought the cow looked quite happy and contented as she lay there warm and protected, chewing her cud. I could hear the grating of the snow as a cruel wind drove it over the roof past the hole, and knew it was below zero up there. It was a strange kind of stable, but the cow did not seem to mind, and submitted to being milked in a calm manner, quite like any other cow. Although she had no exercise, she seemed quite healthy. Tom carried a half pail of milk up the ladder, and then we skied back to the camp. I could see the hole in the snow leading to the stable for some distance, and the hot air coming out of it in the zero weather made a kind of mist, as if smoke were coming from the stable.

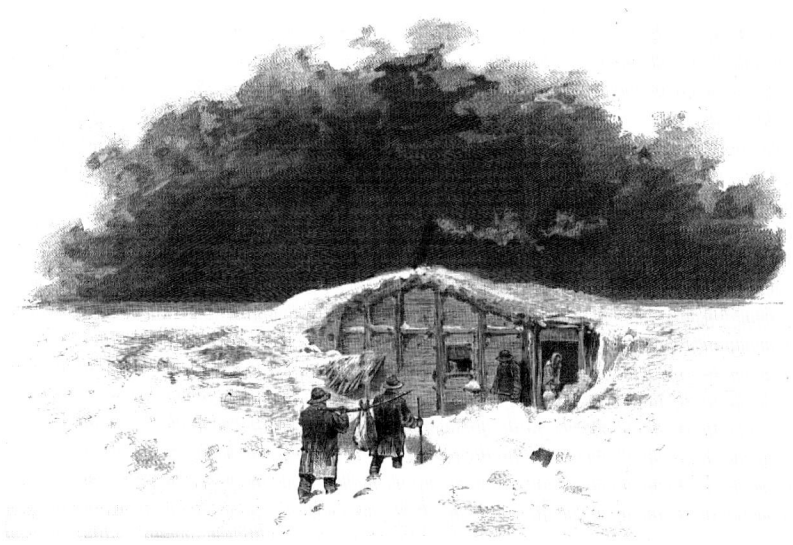

I had forgotten about this cow and her curious stable when, some months later, just before spring opened, I noticed Tom and another man come up out of the hole in the roof and start skiing in a great hurry for Tom's home. I thought nothing of it at the time. The next morning Tom, evidently worried, came over to see me, and told me it was about his cow. It appeared that the cow was about to have a calf, and for two days he had been in the stable most of the time, doing what he could for her. Several cattlemen who were in town had seen the cow, but did not know what the trouble was. The cow was in a bad state. She would not eat or drink, and was suffering a lot of pain. There was some hitch about that calf's coming, and Tom was afraid he might have to shoot the cow if she did not get any better, so he asked me if I would mind coming to see her, for I might know of some way to help her. He said his wife urged him to ask me as she was quite upset over the matter, and the cow was a pet of hers.

Here I was caught again and doing a thing out of my line. I was not brought up on a farm, and all I knew about a cow was that she gave milk. As I climbed down the ladder after Tom into the stable, I was anything but happy in my mind. I had a most vivid picture of how, when I tried to examine her, I would probably get a good hard kick in my stomach. But when in the dim light of the stable I saw the poor creature lying on her side on some hay, I felt only sorrow; she was too weak to kick anyone. There she lay, her brown coat all wet with sweat, her flanks heaving as she panted in short and rapid breaths, her whole body shaking with chills. She gave a low moaning cry as she tossed to and fro in her agony and distress. Her tongue was hanging out, her eyes were bulging, and tears were running down her face. I saw that she was really about to die, and I got to work. I could make out the head of the calf, and it was all bent to one side and stuck fast. I tried to turn it around, but it was like pulling at a rock. I could not move it, for I was not strong enough.

I hated to give up and tell Tom to shoot her. An idea occurred to me. I sent one of the cattlemen who were with us to the general store in town, and he soon came back with a block and tackle used in hauling ore out of a shaft in the mines. I first tied the cow's horns to a log that was part of the manger, so she would not slide along the floor of the stall. Then I lashed the block to one of the posts that held up the roof. I now made a loop in a rope and, after several trials, passed it around the head of the calf. I expected to choke the calf to death, but I did not care. I put the rope through the pulley on the post, and two men stood ready to pull on the rope. All was ready, and I told the men to pull. I guided the head as well as I could by feeling, and I felt it slowly slipping as the rope was pulled taut. Little by little the head was turning. I made the men stop every few minutes, and took my time. At last the calf, a little bull, was born. Wonderful to say, it lived! I had to work over him, pushing his chest in and out, before he could breathe, but at last he gasped, then gave another gasp or so. The poor little thing had been about pulled to pieces, but he was tough. I carried him along to his mother's head, and she very feebly licked him a few times. I knew she would come along all right, with any kind of luck.

So it proved that animals stand such strain far better than human beings do. I suppose they are nearer to nature. As a rule, in animal life, the bearing of offspring is an easy and painless affair. In the case of this particular cow I believe the trouble was probably a lack of exercise.

I always considered that a cow was a most stupid creature, hardly capable of gratitude, and not intelligent enough to remember an act of kindness. I was therefore much impressed by the way this cow acted. Evidently she did remember that I had helped her, because, when I came down the ladder to see her in the stable, she would commence mooing. When I got near her she would lick my hands and clothes, making a funny noise in her throat as if trying to tell me all about it. I was doubtful, and felt she possibly was acting that way with everyone who came near her; but when other men came down to see the calf she grew ugly and tried to horn them. Even Tom, her owner, who milked her and had always handled her, could not touch the calf; she just went wild when he tried to pull the calf away to show it to the people who came down to the stable to see it. Yet I could pull that calf around anywhere, and often picked it up in my arms. She only kept making that queer noise in her throat, and rubbing her head against me.

But the calf was an ungrateful little beast, and when he had grown up to be quite a calf and could frisk all over the stable, I came down the ladder one day to see how he was growing. As

I got off the ladder and took a step on the floor, the little devil suddenly made a rush and gave me a hard butt in the region of my stomach that nearly knocked the breath out of me. After that I carried a stick and gave him a whack to make him more considerate of the doctor who had brought him into the world.

In the spring Tom and his wife moved to another camp, and my cow patient and her bull calf were driven down the valley and out of my life.

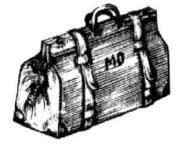

Chapter 2
First Aid Above Timberline

I could hardly realize how deep the snow was until one day I skied over the valley floor. I used my snowshoe pole, seven feet six inches long, and found that in most places I had to push the pole straight down through the snow until my arm was buried to my elbow before I could strike ground. In other places I sat on the tops of telegraph poles where drifts had almost covered them. Of course, snowshoes were worn by everybody. You cannot walk without them through snow that is six to seven feet deep. If you fall off your snowshoes you sink at once out of sight. You struggle up on your feet, the snow up to your chest, and if you struggle much you sink deeper and deeper.

This snow covered the country so deeply that I really hardly recognized it when the spring opened and the snow fields began to sink lower and lower every day. I felt that I was in a new country. As the ground emerged from its blanket of snow, I saw roads I had never heard of, and streams roaring down full of ice. Then came the pattering of rain on roofs. The dripping of water from eaves sounded strange, for no rain ever fell in winter—only snow. The few aspens along the creeks put out some tiny leaves; the sides of the hills showed a little green grass; wild flowers sprang up even near deep snowdrifts.

The whole town began to wake up, like Nature around it, for the short summer. Prospectors and miners were hurrying along the roads and trails to the mines, anxious to get out the ore before the fall arrived with deep snows and cold blizzards, making work above timber line almost too hard to endure. It seemed strange to me to stand on a road and see the six-

First Aid Above Timberline

mule teams clatter and rumble by, the driver shouting, dogs barking, dust, noise, and confusion everywhere; strange too, to remember that only a few weeks before, when I had passed by that exact spot on my snowshoes, there was nothing but a white wilderness of snow. The only sound was the crunch of my shoes on the frozen surface as I glided swiftly and silently along on my rounds with the wind murmuring in my ears, and nothing to see but white snow fields, deep and trackless, and the snow whirling away in spirals from my shoes like a mist as I passed over them. The town itself seemed to wake from a winter sleep. New faces appeared every day. Prospectors and miners now arrived with horses and burros, all intent on reaching the rich lodes of silver ore high up in the mountains to make their fortunes by some lucky strike; ready to risk any dangers and endure any hardships for a chance of success.

It was a novelty to me to see the droves of burros collected in corrals. These donkeys were the only practical way to bring down the ore from the high mines to our camp, and were supposed to be kept in corrals. But many wandered all over the place,

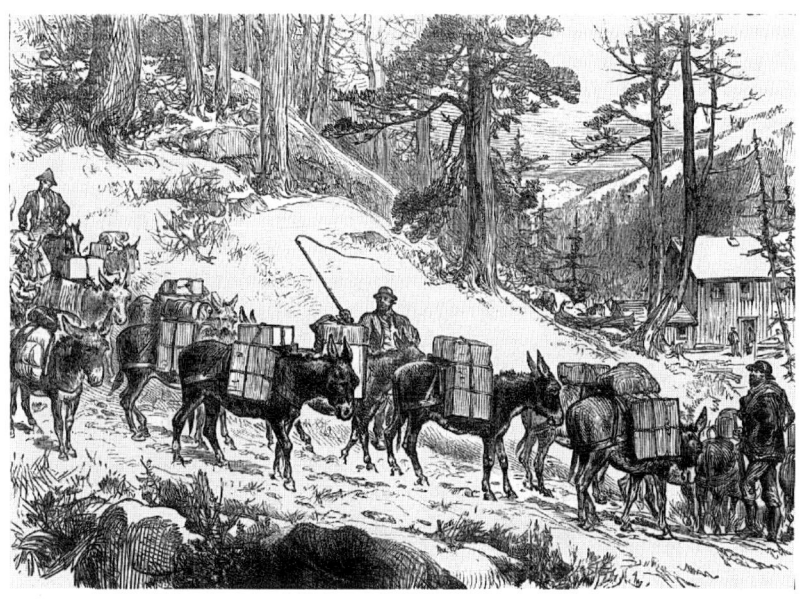

heehawing all night, making love, fighting over garbage, and even trying to eat clothes hung on lines to dry. It was curious to watch them on the narrow trails coming from some mine, laden with ore sacks on their small packsaddles, a long line winding among the rocks and gulches, their long ears pointing forward, their tiny hoofs with little mincing steps going along the very edge of steep cliffs. Led by some wise old veteran, unmoved by storm or wind, slow, sure, patient but obstinate—as his family all over the world—he plodded on, indifferent to abuse or praise. At the end of the string of the tiny cavalcade rode the burro wrangler, astride a bronco. With his pockets filled with rocks, he lounged his slow way along, smoking, half awake. But let a tie-up occur in which the leaders bunched together, crowding on the narrow trail at a bad place where they were uncertain what to do, our sleepy lounger on his horse far back would stand up in his stirrups and, with marvelous accuracy and skill, proceed to "rock" the unfortunate burro who was too stupid to proceed. Soon the long train would be straightened out again, the sacks bobbing back and forth on the backs of the burros at every step down the descent to where at last their packs were taken off to be shipped to the smelter. Later you would see their small legs kicking amid a dust cloud as they rolled their tired and sore backs on the ground.

 From the mountains came the rumble of slides, as this was the time of year when the snows on the mountain sides melted and slid into the valleys. Slides were a real danger on some trails, and so destructive in the spring for a few weeks that no one traveled over these trails. The year before, not two miles up the valley from our town, a bunkhouse at a mine was crushed and carried down to the creek. Without warning, on a night when sixteen miners were asleep in their bunks, a huge slide rushed down the gulch back of the house and across the valley floor, taking the big log bunkhouse with it as if it were made of cards, crushing the big logs like straw, burying it at last under tons of ice and snow. I saw the place with the scattered and splintered logs, pieces of old bedding and clothes, all tumbled around and crushed among the rocks where the poor fellows met their death. All but one were killed. The lone survivor ran two miles in his underclothes in zero weather to our place, arriving half crazy, with frozen hands and feet. A stage with four horses, the driver, and passengers, were caught and buried in a canyon near another camp west of us, and the slide was so deep and frozen so hard that it was late in the fall before the

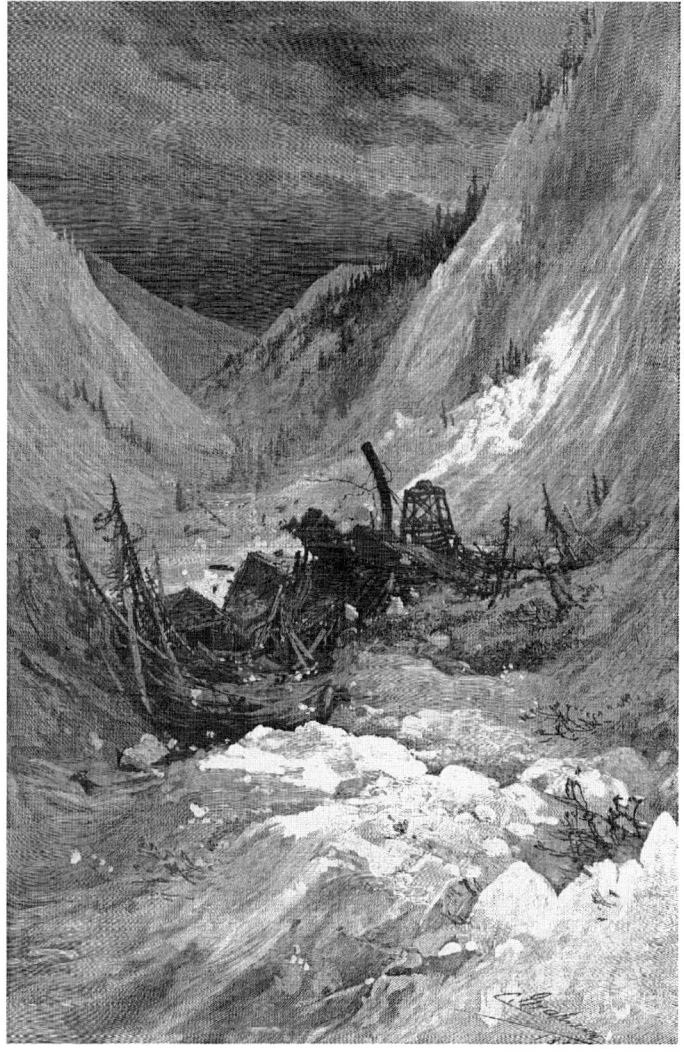

bodies could be dug out. I had never at close quarters actually seen a slide come down. I had seen a path a hundred yards wide down a mountain through big pine and spruce timber, where a slide had broken off the trees three feet from the ground as if some gigantic steam roller had come crashing down, and my fear and respect for their power was very acute. But I was to have a more intimate experience with them.

I was reading in my sleeping room back of my office at about nine o'clock one evening when I heard a knock on my office door. When I got up and opened it, a young fellow I knew by sight half staggered in. I knew he was one of the Wilson boys who had a mine on Black Mountain about fifteen miles north. They were from Ohio, and were fine men, popular, and respected by the camp. As he came in at the door, I first thought this John Wilson was drunk, but as I led him to a chair and he sank into it, I could see that he was tired out. His face, burnt a brick red from the glare of snow fields, was lined with anxiety, and his eyes were sunken with fatigue, making his young face look far older than his years. The way he fell into the chair like a dead man, threw his hat on the floor, and, bending over to the stove for warmth, covering his face with his shaking hands, told only too plainly that some trouble was eating his heart out. He was a big, strong fellow of about my own age, but he shook with cold, and his voice sounded like that of a child as, with faltering words, he tried to tell me his trouble. But I would not let him say another word, for he was too exhausted. He waited while I boiled some coffee and made him eat and drink. Then he briefly told me the trouble he was in.

He was working on his claim with four miners, driving a tunnel into the mountain. It was a wild spot up above thirteen thousand feet. He had brought his younger brother, Tom, out from Ohio with him, and his voice broke as he said, "I promised Mother to look after Tom." The day before, Tom, who was young and reckless, had drilled a hole in the rock at the end of the tunnel they were blasting in the side of the mountain, about forty feet from the entrance. He had put in the powder and fuse and tamped it in, so that when the powder was fired by the fuse the rock would be shattered by the explosion into small enough pieces to be carried out and dumped down the mountain from the mouth of the tunnel.

Tom had lighted the piece of fuse left sticking out of the hole, had watched it sputter and spark as the burning fuse ate its way into the drill hole in the rock, and then had run back to the mouth of the tunnel and outside, where the explosion could not hit him. He had waited a long time, and nothing had happened. At last he had realized that there had been a misfire. The fuse had burned down the hole and gone out before reaching the powder. There was nothing for him to do but drill a new hole or pick out the tamping in the old one, and Tom had gone to work with a steel drill to dig out the small pieces of rock that filled the hole. The rock was hard. The end of the steel drill had struck a spark on the side of the rock inside the hole, set fire to the fuse beyond the place where it had burnt out, and in a flash it had reached the powder. Tom, standing with the drill in his hand, got the explosion right in his face. The other miners were at dinner in the cabin just outside the tunnel. They ran in, and there in the powder smoke they found Tom, his face mashed in, unconscious. They dragged him to the cabin. John, half wild with grief over his brother's injury and suffering, made a fast trip to our camp for a doctor. He had seen the other two doctors: one was too old to stand such a trip up to fourteen thousand feet in deep snow to the mine, while the other had a baby case coming off and could not leave it. So in desperation John had come to me as a last chance.

I told John I would go with him to see his brother. We could not go that night in the dark, but would start the first thing in the morning. John felt better after I promised to go, and went to a room in the hotel for the night. I then packed a small surgical kit in a bag. I knew what a hard trip we should have, so I took only a light outfit. John said he must tell me that the trail up through the gulch to the mine was very dangerous, that slides were running into the creek from the mountains on both sides, and that he had been nearly caught coming down to me. We could ride horses the first part of the way. We then had to go on foot up a canyon on the most dangerous trail in the whole range for slides, and at the worst time of the year for them; climb Black Mountain to fourteen thousand feet, over snow crusted so badly that we could not use snowshoes; then down the other side about two hundred feet to the mine. Fortunately I was in fine condition, as I had been skiing every day. I was as tough as a wolf, and could climb all day.

John came at daybreak with a couple of old saddle horses rented from the livery stable. We rode at a trot along a fair trail for some eight to ten miles, and then entered the deep gulch that was the only way to Black Mountain, a most depressing place. The mountains rose steep and dark on either side in a series of benches; beside us the creek flowed among rocks, the ice still holding it back in places. The whole gulch was still dark in the black shadows of early morning. A keen wind facing us cut like a knife. The trail wound in and out among boulders, at times fifty feet up on the right bank, and then down to the edge of the creek, over the thick ice on the bank, but climbing all the time. Every foot of the way grew rougher. As we rode in single file over the trail through the half-dark before dawn, we said but little. John was worrying about his brother, and I was cold, and anxious over the danger of being caught in a slide. At a turn I caught a first clear view of Black Mountain. Suddenly came a crash like thunder; our horses trembled and stood still; and far up the creek ahead we saw a mass of clouds like snow dust drift over the mountains. We knew a slide had crossed the trail ahead. We looked at each other. Finally John said, "Doctor, I will go ahead a hundred yards and you follow; we must spread out so we can't both be hit."

John went on up the trail, mounting higher and higher up the gulch. I was worried; even my old horse was trembling. At last I could see John far up above me, waving his arm for me to come on. I turned my horse up the bank to a place where it seemed more level. I looked up at the mountain at my right. It was still in deep shadow, but far up where its crest cut the blue sky I saw a gleam of light as the rising sun struck the snow and turned it to gold. That cheered me. It was rough riding on the slippery sidehill. My horse was stumbling, and I was so intent on holding him up I hardly heard a sharp crack from the mountain beside me. Then I heard a deep sound like thunder, and thought another slide was running up ahead. I looked up, and on the side of the mountain right over my head a mass of snow was rolling down straight for me. It came so rapidly, and the crashing roar of it was so confusing, that I had no time to think. A blast of cold wind hit my back, my big hat was blown over my eyes, I felt my horse heave under me as if rearing. Half smothered in snow dust, I felt a blow on my right cheek. I was being rolled over and over—and then I was out of it.

I was lying on cold mud when I felt a stabbing pain in my side, and gasped for breath. I felt of my ribs, and decided I had cracked one. Wet and shivering, I sat up and tried to see where my horse was, but he was out of sight. I fell back in the mud, and was sick. I dug the snow out of my eyes, and finding that my pulse was fair, I just lay quiet for a time, half in a doze. At last a hand caught my coat and shook me, and there was John, out of breath, and calling to me. I could hear nothing, for snow filled my ears. I dug it out, and John was saying, "Are you hurt much, Doctor?" I made an effort and finally told John I was only knocked about a bit and wet from the snow driven into my clothes. I asked to have some whisky, if he could find my bag, which was fastened with straps to my saddle. John went down the bank to the creek where the mass of snow had settled. I could not see it from where I was, but I could hear it crunching and crackling as the heavy wet snow settled into place, and I heard John picking away at something. He was gone a long time, and when he came back he told me my horse was dead and half buried in the frozen slush. John cut away the snow to the cinch of my saddle and there at last found my bag and brought it up to me. Nothing was broken in my bag, and I had a big drink out of my flask. I was not used to it and the whisky just seemed to run all through me. I felt like a new man.

John went back to where he had left his horse up the gulch beyond the slide, brought it back over the trail to where I was, helped me into the saddle, and, leading the horse, we made another mile or so. Here the snow was too deep for the horse, and John turned him back on the trail down the gulch and rocked him a bit with small stones. He made off for home and food. John told me that from his position higher up the gulch and out of the path of the slide, he had seen the slide coming for me, and had a horrible moment as he saw me disappear in the cloud that rolled over the gulch like white smoke. He said that the only thing that saved me was that, just before the slide reached me, it swerved to one side so that I was struck only by the edge where the snow was soft and broken. This snow was only about two feet deep, but it hit the legs of my horse, and he plunged into the deeper part and was carried down, while I was thrown to one side and rolled over and over. I suppose the horse gave me a kick in the side as I fell off him.

We were now well above timber line at the foot of Black Mountain. The slope up to the top was a steep pitch. The snow was only about two feet deep, but was covered with a rough crust. As I looked up and saw how steep and high it was my heart failed me for a moment. The black ridge at the top seemed a long way up in the air. Later in the summer, when the snow melted, there was a burro trail up to the top, but now there was no trail, and the only way up was to kick a hole in the crust at every step, although at every step up we were getting higher, where the thin air was harder to breathe. There was no going back, and the only shelter was the mine over the top on the other side. Where we were the temperature still went to zero every day at sunset. There was no wood for a fire at night, and we should freeze to death unless we could reach the mine. I was feeling pretty bad. My hands were raw, for the slide had scraped the skin off, and my side was stabbing me at every breath, but John Wilson was a prince of a man and, with a touching unselfishness, insisted upon going ahead, carrying my bag and breaking a trail for me to follow. In bad places he held my hands and pulled me up. We could make only a few steps, and then sink down on the snow, gasping for breath.

It was a long tug, and, but for John's help, I could not have done it. I did my best to keep cheerful, and I remember we joked and made light of it all, but I felt like the devil all the way up.

At last we threw ourselves down on the black rocks at the top, all in. On every side there was a glorious view, for we could see miles of high mountain peaks and deep canyons. I am a lover of the mountains, and such a wonderful view was worth going a long way to see. But I had no energy left to enjoy the scenery at an altitude of fourteen thousand feet. The wind was blowing in fierce gusts that sent the cold air through my wet clothes as if they were paper, and all I wanted was to be where I could be safe and warm. The slope to the top of Black Mountain, which we had just climbed through the snow, ended in a long rocky ridge forming the top at fourteen thousand feet. I could now see the other side of the mountain for the first time. There was no snow slope on this other side. The rocky ridge at the summit ended in a cliff which dropped down one thousand feet. I looked over the edge of this cliff, and there, about one hundred feet below us, were the cabin and mine. There was a ledge of rock running down and across the face of the cliff to the cabin, but most of it had been cut into the rock, and even then it was so narrow and partly overhung by the rocks overhead that the only way to go along this trail was to crawl along it on hands and knees.

The cabin was built partly on a ledge of rock, but at least half of it was hanging out over the edge of the cliff. Held in place by logs anchored in holes in the cliff, and by big ropes fastened to iron staples above and on both sides, this cabin looked to me from above like a bird cage tied to a wall. I wondered that a strong wind had not carried it away long before.

The cabin and mine were unusual. I never saw another mine like it in all the years I passed in the mining country. It really was not a mine at all, but a prospect hole these miners had blasted into the mountain in the hope of cutting into a vein of rich ore they had discovered on top of the mountain. It was a desperate attempt to make a fortune, in a time when silver mining was booming. No one but such hardy and reckless men as these early prospectors would have dreamed of building a cabin in such a situation. Everything had to be packed in on men's backs over that narrow ledge. One miner had fallen off this ledge and been killed, but nothing stopped these skillful, strong, and brave men. They would endure any danger or hardship if they saw a chance of grasping a fortune from fate.

John and I lay on that ridge on top, the wind so strong that John had to shout to me, "Put some sand in your coat pockets, Doctor, and throw it along the trail where there is ice."

So I loaded up with a rough sort of sand that was lying in the rock hollows near us, found the beginning of the trail to the cabin, and crawled along it. To say I was fearful of falling off is to put it mildly. I was in a blue funk. My nerves were ragged, anyway, and my side hurt me with every breath I took. I dared not look over the edge at my left that went down straight one thousand feet. The wind was howling around me, trying to push me over and, as a last straw, I was having mountain sickness because of the altitude.

Good old John came on behind me, and I threw sand on the trail before me where the drip from the cliff above had

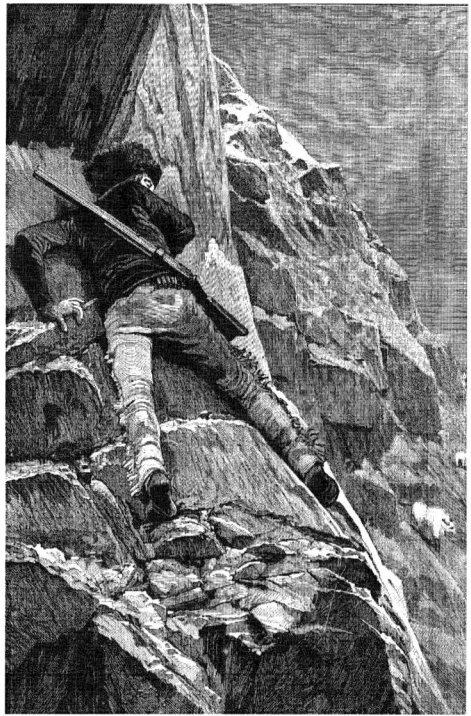

frozen into hummocks I had to crawl over. About halfway to the cabin a little gully crossed the trail, and here a stone about the size of a baseball came tumbling down, hit the ice between my hands on the trail in front of my face, and bounded off again, spattering my face with ice water. Off my guard, I jerked back. My left knee suddenly slipped from under me, my body slued around, and my leg was over the edge. I dug my fingernails into the ice, my right knee gritted on the sand a bit and then held fast as I slowly pulled my leg back, leaning all my weight against the wall on my right. I heard John behind me saying, "Gosh, that was a close one." Then my nerves gave way, and in a panic I scrambled recklessly along, not looking ahead, my eyes on the rocky trail under me.

I did not know where I was until suddenly strong hands caught my coat and I was lifted to a platform by the cabin, where the miners had been watching me. I fainted as they carried me into the cabin, but came to in a few minutes, and these miners got to work. They stripped me, wrapped me in warm blankets, put a hot stove lid wrapped in newspapers at my feet, dosed me with whisky and rubbed my thin body with their rough hands until I felt on fire all over. I fell asleep, and when I woke up I looked around the cabin. The walls and ceiling, dingy from smoke, were built of rough boards, and pictures from the *Police Gazette*—or some such source—were tacked up on the walls. A string held some very dirty socks hanging up to dry, and from pegs hung coils of rope, old slickers, and caps. The floor was all mud and dirt, cluttered with drills, sledges, rubber boots, and a small grindstone. A table standing in the middle of the room had boxes for seats. Bunks were built against the wall on one side, and a cookstove that was roaring—the crazy stovepipe leaking smoke at every joint—completed the furnishings of the room. When the wind struck the cabin it creaked and groaned like a ship at sea, and the ropes holding it to the cliff sang like violin strings as they caught the strain.

A man was bending over the stove, cooking, and I could smell flapjacks and bacon grease. I heard a man moaning and turning in the bunk next to me, but I could not see him. The man at the stove filled a cup with water and went over to the sufferer. I heard choking sounds as he tried to swallow. Then the man with the cup came back to the stove, put the cup on a shelf, spat on the floor, and said, "Christ, this sure is hell!"

I knew then that my patient Tom was in the bunk. John came in. "Can you get up, Doctor? I want you to see my brother." John helped me dress. I was shaky, but got to work. The details are too horrible to relate. I dressed the poor boy's face, taking out pieces of rock. He was blind and quite deaf from the blast, and burned from the powder flash. I gave him a big hypodermic of morphia and, thank Heaven, it worked, so that after an hour he lay in a kind of stupor, but free from pain for the first time since he was hurt.

We had supper—the same old beans, bacon, and dough bread that was the usual meal in camps, varied occasionally by dried apples, potatoes, or flapjacks. I here saw for the first time beans being baked in an altitude kettle. At thirteen thousand feet you cannot boil potatoes or beans as you can at sea level; the water boils hard enough, but the air is so thin it all boils away without getting hot enough to cook beans or potatoes. So a boiler is used with the lid clamped down so that the boiling is done under pressure. There is a safety valve so that the steam blows off if the pressure becomes too high.

After supper I told John we must carry Tom down to town at a lower level, for his wounds were infected, and I feared pneumonia at that high altitude. We finally made a sled on which to lift him down over the snow on the other side. We put four skiis together, side by side, and fastened them by nailing pieces of board across to hold them in place. Then I went to bed, and the miners played freeze-out poker on the table. They were a hard-looking lot, with beards and long hair. They were spattered from head to foot with mud, for the tunnel where they worked dripped water all over them. Their language was profane, to say the least, while they shouted with delight at the vilest stories I ever heard. All the time they chewed and spat tobacco juice on the floor, telling one another what a real spree they would have if they did strike it rich. I was so disgusted I rolled over in my bunk so that I could not see them.

I was to have another scare from the mountain that night. The cabin was built at a place where there was a crack in the cliff above it, and rocks pried out by the frost kept falling down on the roof. Before they hit the roof you could hear them crack loose from the cliff above and come rolling down. If the noise they made was very loud and a big one was coming, someone yelled "Tunnel!" and everyone had time to run into the tunnel where he could be safe if the cabin was carried away.

Fortunately this alarm was given only twice. The first time the rock missed the cabin and went crashing down the cliff to one side. The other time it struck the roof a terrible blow. The logs on the roof cracked, and the old cabin rocked and shivered as if it would fall to pieces. But it held, and the men came back from the tunnel, cold, wet, and joking about it. I stayed in my bunk, too tired to care much, and poor Tom was so doped he never woke up.

At daylight the miners got busy and prepared to take Tom over the trail to the snow fields on the other side. I was worried by the thought of carrying Tom over that rock trail along the face of the cliff. It was all a man could do to go over it alone, and carrying a man in Tom's helpless condition seemed a great risk. I was too knocked about by the slide the day before to help much, but these miners were equal to anything, and were used to carrying over this trail. Tom was in bad condition. He had a high temperature, blood poisoning, and was very weak. I had him all bandaged up for the trip and gave him another hypodermic of morphia so he might not suffer by the jolting he was bound to get. These miners made the trail ready for carrying Tom over it by chipping all the ice away so there would be less danger of stepping over the cliff. They could not use the sled we had made out of skis, for the trail was too narrow. So they put Tom on a piece of canvas held together at the top, something like a hammock, and a man at each end half lifted and half dragged Tom along this narrow path to the snow.

At last we were all over, and Tom was on the sled. We now had to go down two thousand feet over a snow field that was at an angle of forty-five degrees. The snow had a crust on it too rough to ski over, but the sled could slide down while we held it back by ropes. To do this, since the slope was so steep, we had to kick a hole in the crust to get a foothold, let the sled down a few feet, and then kick through the crust again. Very hard work it was! The sled, with poor Tom helpless on it, tugged on the ropes, and the men held back for dear life. If the sled got away on that incline, it was good-by to Tom, for nothing could save him. He would be dashed into the gulch below us.

Every now and then someone would slip, trying to hold the sled back, and slide under the crust on his back, to come up blowing and half smothered. All the boys worked with wonderful spirit, joking and keeping our spirits up, and at last, tired and hot, we arrived at the base and commenced going down the gulch where I had been hit by the slide. Here we had to carry Tom on the sled, for there was no snow. John hurried on ahead and came back with a bunch of prospectors. Everyone took hold, and we made good time. We feared slides, but none came our way. We passed the place where I had been tumbled about the day before. The creek was dammed up by the snow, and out of the frozen mass the hind legs of my unfortunate horse stuck up stiffly, a mute reminder of the danger I had been in. We got the saddle, and a miner carried it on his shoulders the rest of the way. I hurried by this place, for it gave me the creeps to look up at the mountains on each side, fearful lest another slide come down. A little farther on I looked back to see the last of Black Mountain with its dark top ridge in a haze of snow smoke.

Before me a trail wound along by the half-frozen creek. The gulch was dark and cold, and the figure on the frail sled rocked and pitched as my good friends, the miners, carried it down the rocky and rough trail with constant care and tenderness. Some prospectors joined us and helped carry Tom, and then, at last, we were on the road in an ore wagon that took us all to town.

I dressed my patient's wounds again and arranged with his brother John to start for Denver in the morning, in the hope that an oculist might possibly save his sight. I never saw them again, but John wrote me that poor Tom's eyes were destroyed beyond repair.

That night I fell asleep, worn out, only to wake up towards daylight with a severe attack of blood poisoning. My arms were swollen; I had a high fever, and was out of my head for ten days. My hands were skinned when the slide rolled me over, and I suppose some pus got on them when I was dressing the wounds on Tom's face up on Black Mountain. Some of the boys sat up day and night and nursed me, and I recovered.

Chapter 3
My Dream Horse

As a frontier doctor, I had to make long trips to see my patients, sometimes one hundred and thirty miles, along faint trails, hard to follow, with but very few ranches for stopping places. When the rivers were up and fords too deep, I had to swim my horse across. When I was called on these trips, you may be sure it was no fancied illness, but something serious, that demanded all the speed I could make. There was, in fact, very little illness among the hardy cattle men and women who took up ranches in those days, and most of my calls were to treat injuries, such as gunshot or fractures, so that I had to go, night or day, storm or calm. As I was obliged to go in the shortest possible time and, of course, on horseback, the main thing was to have a good horse—one that you could trust on a narrow, dangerous trail, that was good in rapid water, and above all, so tough he could keep going for fifty or sixty miles and, even in hobbles, eat enough grass at night to be able to go on again the next day.

At that time the half-wild native horse, called the bronco, was the only one that could stand the pace and exposure. Many horses were better bred, were larger and finer-looking, and could travel faster for a time. But to endure cold and heat, to keep going on only grass for food, day after day, without shelter at night, pawing through snow to get a little cured grass underneath, in zero weather and biting wind, the bronco, as used by the cowboys to drive cattle, was the only breed to use.

I had a corral near my house and owned three or four broncos which were good, as they go. I fed them a little grain to keep them up, but none of them was to be trusted. As I came in from a long ride, tired out, looking forward to a good dinner and restful night, often, on my doorstep would sit a cowboy. As I came up he would say something like this, "Say, Doc, I came from Abe Buford's place. His wrangler has got throwed and busted his leg; he sure needs you bad, Doc."

So I must saddle a fresh horse and start on another thirty miles or so. Often, being tired and careless, I would swing into the saddle, and then, my new mount being fresh, there would be "crowhopping" that jarred my tired bones to the limit before I could get him into a lope. At such times I often indulged in daydreams, when I pictured to myself how nice it would be if somehow I could find the ideal horse I often thought about. He must be a horse that would be gentle-gaited, one that I could talk to, a companion in my long and lonely rides; one that I could trust, and that would be kind and tough; a horse I could guide with my knees; that would stop at a word, follow me like a dog, lie down at command, and guard me when I was asleep. I had read of such horses among the Arabs, but it was all a dream, I knew, although I had thought about it so much I could see him plainly in my mind's eye. How he stood looking at me with his kind, intelligent eyes! How strong and straight his legs were, and how his coat shone in the sun! How I would pet him, I thought, if I had him!

I was not thinking about my dream horse one morning as I rode along the trail up the river. I was going to see a man at the Z. O. Ranch, some fifteen miles above us. This man had, by accident, shot himself through the foot with a big Colt revolver, and his foot and leg were in a terrible state. I was thinking this morning what more I could do to help him when I noticed a dust cloud on the trail some way ahead. I pulled up to see what it was. It looked to me as though a couple of bulls were fighting. It was not moving along the trail. After a bit I went on and soon saw what it was. A bronco was on the trail, kicking and rearing; two men I knew had their ropes on him, one in front and one in back. Every now and then the wild bronco would make a rush at one of the men, and the other man would set his horse back, holding him by his rope, so the bronco could not reach either, no matter how he lunged. Cowboylike, the two were laughing and, as I rode nearer, one of them called out, "Look out, Doc, don't crowd him none; we sure got a bad one here. Talk about your outlaws! This bird bit the pants off Charlie Green last night and would a-killed him only I got my rope on him and threw him by a front foot. We tried every way to gentle him, but he's sure a wildcat. The boss told us to drag him to town and sell him for five dollars or trade him for a few drinks, anyhow."

I just sat my horse and watched this wild bronco. He was quiet for a time and, as my eyes ranged over him, I saw his small head, thick neck, straight legs, and large, intelligent eyes. As I saw his coat glisten in the sunshine like copper, my heart gave a thump! Why, here was my dream horse come to life, right before me in the flesh! I could hardly believe it, but there he was just as I had pictured him in every line of his body. As I sat watching him, he suddenly became ugly, bared his teeth, reared, beating the air with his front hoofs, and made a rush as quick as lightning at one of the men holding him. But the boys were ready, and the rope pulled him back. No matter how savagely he lunged, he was held, and little by little he was being forced along the trail. Again he was quiet a moment, only his head shaking as if saying, "No! No!" He was a beauty, if only he were tame. The idea came to me like a flash—why not buy him and see what kindness can do?

As if in answer to my thought, Charlie, one of the wranglers, said, "Say, Doc, if that bronc could be gentled he'd sure be the best cow horse in the country!"

My mind was made up. I called out, "If you fellows will put him in my corral, I'll buy him right now."

That raised a laugh, of course, but finally I gave them five dollars and went on my way. Looking back along the trail after a mile or so, I could see a dust cloud and knew that the battle was still going on. When I had made my call and reached home, all was quiet at the corral. I could see a few men sitting on the top rail, and from the remarks I could overhear, my captive was at least creating some interest in town. As I came up to the corral, the crowd greeted me, "Oh, Doc, go in and take his temperature." Or, "Go on in and ride him," all with much good nature, yells, and laughter. Occasionally a man would make as if to drop down inside, and then my bronco, roused to fury, would charge the man, and as his tormenter climbed to safety, would dash at the stout logs, kicking and biting the bark off in his frenzy. After a time, the crowd grew tired and left us in peace.

It was lucky that my corral was made of heavy logs. Even then the whole thing would shake when my bronco beat against it; but I knew it was safe, as I had made it to hold hay and keep out stray cattle that would wander down from the hills at night during the winter and try to tear the corral to pieces to get at the hay, so fierce were they from hunger.

In the morning I found my bronco as full of fight as ever, and I had my doubts about how to begin my taming tactics. I could not get near the corral. He acted like a freshly caged tiger. I threw over a forkful of hay, and he kicked and stamped on it like a crazy creature. And yet, as I looked at this wild creature, my heart was full of sympathy; he was not to blame. He had been free and happy running over the wide prairies, and then, suddenly, hateful men had thrown a rope that choked off his breath as it grew tighter and tighter around his neck, until he fell down, so weak he could not fight back. They had tied him, and then, when he grew stronger, and struggled, they had beaten him on the head until, crazed by fear and hatred, he had become a wild beast. He would kill and never give up. His proud spirit could not be broken; he would die first, and his splendid strong body, active as a mountain lion's, matched his brave heart. That is how I understood him and, thinking this over as I walked around, at a loss what to try next, I was joined by an old patient of mine, called "Dutch Charlie," a queer character who lived in a shack all alone and owned a few head of stock. A dirty, drunken old cattleman he was, but wise in his own way, and devoted to me, for I had cured him of a chronic malaria of many years' standing.

Dutch came riding up on his old cow pony and, getting off with a grin of welcome, he pointed to my bronco and said, "Is that the spoilt horse you was calculating to break?"

"Yes," I replied, "and it looks like a hard job for a doctor, doesn't it?"

"Well, I don't know, Doc. You ain't fit to go wrangling with him. He'll sure as hell kill you before you've half gentled him. I'll tell you, Doc, what you do. You just cut out his feed and water until he's that weak he can't stand, and then water and feed him kind of gentle, stroking him and talking to him like he was a human, and if you don't kill him a-doing it, he maybe will come gentle." And then old Dutch Charlie rode off without another word.

It was an idea new to me, but I started right away. A little irrigation ditch ran through one side of the corral where stock could water. This I turned aside so that there was no water in the corral. Then I just waited two days. My dream horse was as ugly as ever, but growing thin and weak. A few days more and my bronco was a sick horse. He had been given no food at all, and only a little moisture from the damp ground along the bottom of the old ditch had he taken. He was eating this dirt; he was shaky on his legs, trembled at times, and his breath rattled in his throat. Still he gave me wicked looks, and I dared not go into the corral.

In the morning, just at daylight, my bronco was down, lying on his side. At first I thought I had gone too far and he was dead, but, looking more closely, I could see his flanks heaving faintly as his breathing lifted them. I was afraid he would die, and I felt ashamed of myself. I had made this poor creature suffer without reason. I blamed myself for not shooting him at first. Full of remorse, I let down the bars and went inside. I was still not sure of him, and with a revolver in one hand I pelted him with some chips of wood. Then I walked nearer and poked him with a stick. He didn't notice me. But I was taking no chances with this animal. He might come around, I thought. Suddenly a wave of compassion came over me, and I felt that I must help him at any risk. I was alone, and was tempted to call some of the boys to help me. But, no, I would treat him and see it through. I ran for a pail of water, dashed into it a bottle of whisky, and knelt down by the horse. I need not have been fearful. The splendid vitality and the wild anger were gone. As I lifted his head he gave me a look out of his softened eyes like a sick baby. Right then I felt he was mine, and I determined to save him if I worked day and night.

I ran a little water and whisky into his mouth, but he could not swallow; I held his head in my lap and massaged his throat until, choking and coughing, he swallowed some water. Then I ran to my haystack and piled all I could under him. The ground was cold, so I half covered him with the hay. As I came and went, his eyes followed me with pathetic helplessness.

I carried my breakfast to his side and ate it there, huddled up by him so as not to lose a moment. I worked all day over him, rubbing him and dropping whisky down his throat. That night I built a campfire in the corral to warm myself and my patient as I sat out the long hours. The next day he was better,

My Dream Horse

breathing more easily, and I fed him a warm mash. Some of the boys came over from town and, after a few sarcastic jokes, entered into the spirit of the thing. They helped me roll him over on some fresh hay, and rubbed him all over.

Another day and night went by. Soon I knew that the crucial moment had arrived. As he got stronger, what would happen? Would all his old anger and aversion to man break out again? I was worried about this. I kept talking to him and rubbing him with my hands. He could now eat all right, and move his head and legs, and I had some anxious moments as to how soon he would remember, and suddenly snap a finger off or kick me when I was not watching.

I was foolish to worry. His devotion was touching. He would not let me leave him, but would raise his head and whinny for me to come back, and then smell my clothes all over to be sure I was there. It was embarrassing, for at night he called for me and struggled, trying to get up. Finally I had to light my lantern and go down and sit by him to comfort him as if he were a frightened child. Before long he could stand up and walk with stumbling steps about the corral. I tried him out by pulling his tail and ears, lifting all his feet a little, and slapping him all over. He just nosed me and bit my coat a little in play. My joy was great. I had won out by kindness when he was weak. This man-killer had become as tame as a collie dog. As day by day he grew stronger, I watched his returning beauty. The silk coat shone; the muscles rippled when he moved with quick and tiger-like grace. He was a splendid animal—my dream horse coming to life!

But there was one fly in the ointment: he was as gentle as a lamb, and a nice pet, but of no use to me. I must have a horse I could ride in my work, and here the real trouble came in; I was still afraid of him, of what would happen when I was in a saddle on his back. There was no telling, and I had a vivid picture of how he could buck if he wanted to.

Well, I had to begin, and this is how I managed it: I had first to get him used to a bridle or, at least, to a rope around his neck. I used a rope, but only a short piece, and there was a circus! He reared and fell over, then scraped his neck against the rough logs of the corral, and it was a good hour before I could get near enough to cut the rope off. He was sweating and trembling all over, and finally came to me for help. I had been too fast. He remembered how he had been nearly strangled to death by the cowboys when they roped him. I now carried a bit of rope on my shoulders, let him smell it, rubbed it gently against him, got him used to it day by day. I put it gently on his back, then on his neck; at last I tied it on his neck and left it there, where he wore it for a week. Then I led him by it. At last I took a turn around his mouth, always slowly and gently, and at last the bridle was worn. Then I tied him to a post, and he understood. I used a stick in his mouth at first, and then a regular bit, and taught him to turn, to stop, to obey the bit and reins.

Now came the saddle. I put a saddle in the corral, placing his oats upon it so he had to feed all over it and turn it over to get oats from underneath. I lifted the saddle and put it gently on his back. Then I cinched it on him loosely, every day cinching it a little tighter. Even then I was afraid to get into the saddle. Not only that, but if he got ugly or frightened at this stage and bucked me off, he was, I felt, an outlaw again. So I filled a sack with sand, a long sack tied in the middle, that hung down on each side of the saddle as my legs would, and was about my weight. To my surprise he didn't do a thing but look at me as if to ask "What are you doing all this for?" After several days of this I left the sack on him all day.

At last I got my courage up. I must ride him, and the

My Dream Horse

ground was pretty soft, anyway. So, my knees trembling, I very slowly and gently mounted him, kicked my feet clear, and put one hand on the saddle horn so I could push back and fall off easily at the first buck. To my surprise nothing happened! He just walked and trotted around that corral as if he had been ridden by children all his life. I could hardly believe it, and when I got down I almost kissed him, I felt so glad and happy. I had won out, but I was conscious that I did not want any mistakes or to have the laugh of the town at the "Doc's bronco busting." I therefore rode him at dusk down to a little meadow near the river where none of the boys could see me, and then I made him lope figure of eights, turn short around trees, guide by knee pressure, stop dead at a word, and so forth. He was splendid! He took to cow-pony tricks like anything and seemed to enjoy it.

He was anxious to be with me at all times, and followed me around like a dog. When I made him stand and wait for me until I was out of sight, then called, he came running after me. Soon he understood the whistle and, if he was confined in any way by a fence, he broke through or jumped over it.

I had been caught pretty badly a year before when I was riding a mean bronco through down timber. As he stumbled and fell, my foot caught in the stirrup, and I was thrown onto my back in a bad position. The beast plunged to his feet and kicked at me as I dragged behind him. He soon got tangled up in some dead timber, and I got out with some bad bruises; so I was rather fearful of being caught by my dream horse in this way.

I therefore trained him not to kick at anything at any time. I did it by filling an old bag about four feet long with old clothes in imitation of a man. This bag I tied to one stirrup by a rope just long enough to drag the end of the bag on the ground and have it pound along, striking his heels at every step. I led him out into the middle of the corral and let go the bag when he was trotting beside me. Then things happened all at once. Amid kicking, squealing, and bucking, the bag was soon torn to pieces, and old clothes and bits of bag were scattered all over the place. It cost me a week and many bags to quiet his fear, but in the end, when the bag was let go and it bumped his legs, he just stood still. It was lucky I had taught him this trick, because later I was thrown when he came down on ice; my foot caught so fast I could not get it out of the stirrup; and my dream horse stood like a rock until I reached up and managed to untie the cinch. The saddle dropped off, and I pulled my foot out of the stirrup, which had been so twisted that it held my foot like a vise.

 The training was over; and now the time had come for me to show him off before the cowboys and ride down the main street. I knew I was in for a lot of fun. The cowboys knew that I was trying to break an outlaw, but I kept pretty dark about it, and only one or two suspected that I had succeeded. Of course the minute they saw me riding down the street, they would try to scare my horse, all in good nature. You see, here was a doctor invading their special work, and to get him thrown and take the conceit out of him was only natural. I chose the noon hour when everybody was lounging around on the wooden sidewalk waiting for the dinner bell. I came trotting down the street, my beauty stepping in little hops. One fellow raised the long yell, and out from the stores and saloon came the crowd, yelling, firing their pistols in the air, and shying their hats under my horse. He never minded a bit. They yelled, "Stick him, Doc, and make him buck." One wrangler, Tom Logan, from the L. O. T. outfit, was on his horse, and a little drunk, so he came and tried to ride us off into the ditch. I could not do anything, for Tom was a good sort and only meant a bit of fun, but my horse, still savage about other men, turned like a fury and bit Tom's pony in the ear and then grabbed Tom's knee in his teeth and nearly had him off before I managed to pull my horse back. The boys had a fine laugh at Tom over this, but soon they went in to dinner, so it came off all right. A few came up to me and called out, "You done fine, Doc! Who is you going to wrangle for now?"

 After this I had all the comfort on long and difficult trails I had often imagined. His gait was a soft fox trot that ate up the distance without tiring man or horse; he was fast and quick when needed, and many a long ride I had on him. In water he had the cool caution that is natural to broncos, picking his way over rocks on the bottom, leaning against the current, keeping to the ford with a kind of instinct, and, on one occasion, crossing Bear River in the winter. It was a stretch of some two hundred yards; ice cakes were coming down with the current, and the air was about zero. He was carried off his feet, and away we went, the banks sliding past us and the current turning us end for end. I was worried, but my dream horse just took it calmly. He swam deeply and carefully, and finally we landed on a sandy bank, half a mile below.

I never could break him of his fear of others. This trait made him difficult to manage. It often happened that, after making a call on some patient at a ranch miles away, some of the boys would show up on the trail home, driving a bunch of cattle. By a natural custom of the country, I at once started in to round up the strays and help them out. At such times my bronco was all interest, running and turning steers with the best cow pony of the outfit. But once we camped and any men came near him, he was all for war at once, showing his teeth and trying to strike. At last I had to warn everyone to keep away from him.

This wildness of his nearly got me into a serious scrape one day. I was up the river at the L. O. T. Ranch to see a cowboy called Sam Clark. Clark had been thrown and tangled up in a barbwire fence, and was torn up pretty badly. As I rode up to the bunkhouse there were a few of the boys just sitting up against the house waiting for dinner. I got off and threw my reins down some way off, so my bronco would not make trouble. All said, "Howdy, Doc," but one little wrangler called "Ginger," who thought he would be smart, said, "Say, Doc, I hear you got a wild one there. I guess you have the crowd buffaloed. I bet I could handle him."

I just said, "You leave him alone, Ginger," and went into the cabin where poor Sam, in a bunk, was waiting for me.

I was getting some hot water ready when I heard a row outside. I jumped to the door, and there was Ginger running around the only tree in sight, and right on his heels was my bronco, snapping and trying to strike him. They were whirling around the tree so rapidly and raising such a lot of dust it was hard to see them. Ginger had had his shirt bitten from his shoulder, and was yelling "Shoot him! Shoot him!" I ran to them, caught my bronco, and stopped him. Ginger, in a rage, his face white as a shirt, grabbed a gun out of the belt of one of the men, and in a moment would have killed my horse. I didn't think of consequences, but drew my gun and covered Ginger. Immediately several of the boys jumped in and tore our guns away from us. It all happened in a second, and I was lucky, for Ginger was a bad actor, had killed a man the fall before at Red Mountain and, no doubt, would have killed me before I could shoot. At last we all had a peace talk, which ended by Ginger's riding into town with me. Ever after we were the best of friends.

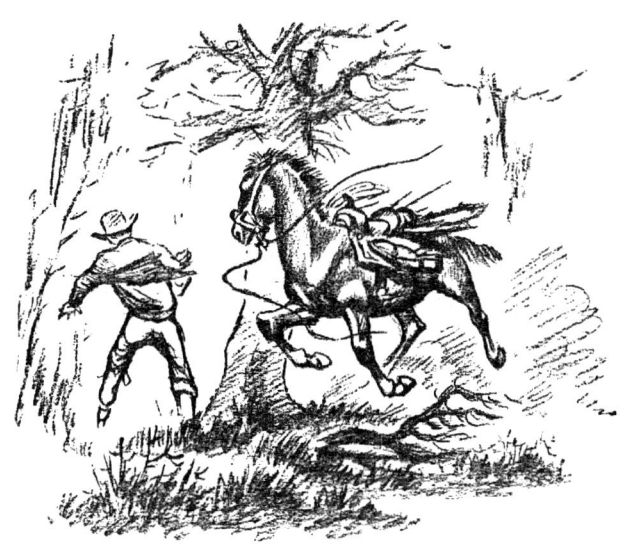

Chapter 4
The Widow's Herd

Our little town was all set for the spring roundup. Some sixty cattlemen were riding out. All had a few cattle that had been running on the open range during the winter, for there were no fences in those days. Every spring and fall we rounded up all the cattle on the river and back in the hills into one big herd, cut out the calves and beef cattle, branded the calves, and drove the beef cattle two hundred miles to the railroad. Then we let the rest scatter on the range again.

We did things in order, and the first thing was to elect a captain of the roundup whose word was law. Much depended on the captain. Generally elected by popular vote, he was a man who knew the cattle country, especially that part of the open range where we were. It was agreed that the captain had to be an old hand, who knew the cattle business and so could work his men with a system; and, above everything else, he must be a man liked and trusted by the boys—a man to depend upon to have a nerve of iron when necessary. Such a man we had this spring in Charlie Thompson, a fine type of cattleman who knew his business and was respected by all.

"Doc," Charlie said to me, "why don't you come along with us on the roundup? Ain't hardly nobody left in town, and if the boys get hurt, you'll be handy. You can ride your own horse and sling your bedroll in the wagon." So I went with the outfit, a kind of cowboy surgeon, for six weeks. I took my surgical instruments and my rifle and had some fine hunting, but there was little medical practice, for the boys were as hard as nails.

As we rode out of town we were, I suspect, a wild-looking lot; the mess wagon lumbered along, driven by Charlie, a darky cook; then the bunch of extra broncos herded by the horse wranglers in a cloud of yellow dust; and, above all, the men who drove the cattle, all armed with rifle and revolver.[1] Why? In a roundup where I was in early days, the men were forced to scatter over a wild and rough country; often they killed game for food. But above all, men were away from the main camp for days at a time. Often it was on the cards to see cattle and horse thieves making off with your cattle, and you must be able to guard your property. The boys did not pack guns because they wanted to kill anyone, but because if well armed they would not be an easy mark for the outlaws who preyed on the weak and the defenceless, rather than on the outfits well armed and prepared to defend themselves and their property.

A young fellow rode with us, a tenderfoot as green as paint, but treated kindly by the boys because, as one expressed it, "He was so d—— innocent." This boy had arrived in town some months before, driving a couple of skin-and-bone animals that were hardly able to drag the old wagon, which was all tied up with baling wire, and wobbling all over the road. The boy, with his red, innocent, sunburnt face and big blue eyes, walked by the wagon, while in the wagon, tired and weary, sat a slip of a girl, a kind of weak, faded blonde (only a child she seemed to us), and in her arms was a little baby whom she rocked up and down as it cried. Covered with dust, clothes ragged, they had come all the way from Carolina to make their fortune in Colorado. This family came to a halt in front of Mother White's Hotel, and out came Mother White. We men held back, while Mother White settled these penniless children in a little shack.

Mother White had had a stormy past, and rumor had it that morals were not respected by her to any marked degree. But when I saw her hard face soften and tears drop from her eyes as

---

[1] It may seem strange in this day when all the Western country is settled up, to speak so often of the cowboys going out on their business armed with rifle and revolver. More than once I have heard men say, "I never carried a weapon in my life, and I rode all over the West and never had any trouble. It was really safer to go unarmed." No doubt, among bad men in saloons and dance halls, a stranger was better off without a gun. On the open range it was different.

she held the little baby she took from the tired mother, I felt that possibly Mother White's sins were forgiven her. At any rate, we all helped the family along, and when the roundup was due, the boy, whose name was Dick Murphy, nearly plagued the life out of Charlie Thompson for permission to come on the roundup with us and learn all about the cattle business. When Murphy's wife chimed in, Charlie yielded. The boy was no help, of course. He had no cattle and no horse, except one of the old horses he drove in with; but nothing mattered as long as he could ride with real cowboys. So he kissed his baby and his crying wife, and came along. We all liked this young fellow, so full of youth and high spirits, so anxious to learn to be a puncher, so willing to laugh at his own mistakes. Then, too, the boys felt sorry for him, so poor and yet so brave in his poverty; I fancy, too, the girl wife and baby, left in town, struck some note in the hearts of these rough men, and they were gentle with the boy on that account. No free lance of the olden time ever rode forth with greater courage and higher hope.

Three days later we were working the slide-rock country down the river, combing the hills and gulches for stray stock. All through this region the foothills were composed largely of loose rocks, which ages ago had slid from the main range. Although these hills were now covered with sage and scrub oak, the gravel underneath was loosely packed, likely to give way under man or horse and slide downhill in a cloud of dust. Consequently, the cowboy had to be careful in riding these slopes, or a bad fall was certain. I got fed up lying around camp all day, talking to black Charlie and reading in the shade of the mess wagon while the boys were out combing the range for cattle, so one morning I rode out, bright and early. The wranglers had brought in my horse "Chum" from the night herd, and I saddled and was off. I wanted to help the boys a little, and while I was not an expert range rider, my bronco was one of the best cattle horses in Colorado and could drive a cow or a wild steer without any help from me; all I had to do was to stick on. We drove a few steers into the herd, and the boys scattered out and left me alone in the hills.

Presently, in a little gulch about four miles from camp, I came upon one crafty old steer that sulked among the scrub oak in the bottom of the gulch and would not move. I got off and rocked him, and soon he was running and snorting down the gulch until, far away from the ridge I was on, I could see some of the boys turning him into the herd collected in the valley below me. I rode the ridge for a time, looking over the country when, about one hundred yards away, on the other edge of the gulch, a steer crashed through the bushes and went tearing down the side of the gulch; after him came two cowboys, swinging their ropes and yelling. One was Dutch, an old hand, and the other rider, I saw, was Dick Murphy, our young novice, riding his old broken-kneed horse, and wild with excitement. Dutch, knowing the risk of a fall, slowed up, but Dick, his old horse

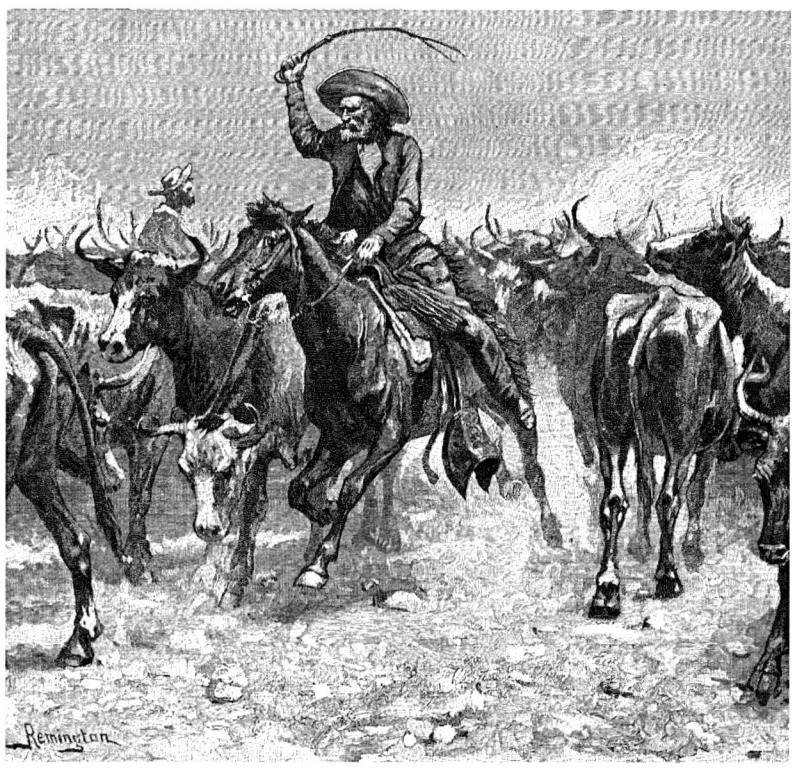

The Widow's Herd

plunging and slipping, went on down a slope full of slide-rock and as steep as a roof.

He was blind, in his excitement, to the dangers of his treacherous footing. I heard Dutch cry out in an effort to stop him, and then it happened all in a bare second. Dick's horse stumbled, half recovered, then, with a crash, man and horse turned a somersault; there was a roar of rocks tumbling down in a cloud of dust. Dick's horse ran loose and riderless down the gulch, and a crumpled figure lay quiet by a scrub oak. I could make out the fair hair on the head in the sunlight. I saw Dutch turn his horse, ride over to the figure, get off, and bend over him; then he saw me and waved for me to come. I hurried over and dismounted, and as I turned the limp body over I could feel the neck bones crunch under my fingers, and I knew that his neck was broken. I tried to make him breathe, but he was dead. Dutch took his hat off and stood a minute in silence, his hard face filled with sorrow, and then he said, "Doc, he's gone. You stay by him while I go to camp for help." I could hear Dutch's horse rattling the loose stones as he rode slowly back to the chuck wagon and main camp down below me in the valley.

All was very quiet and lonely as I covered Dick with my saddle blanket and put his hat over his face. The blue jays chattered and flew from bush to bush; a dead man was nothing in their lives. The sun grew hot as the day wore on; my horse stamped at the flies; the grasshoppers flew past me, making a noise like a rattlesnake. The air was very still and clear. I could see the snowy mountains of the Great Divide far away to the north, glittering in the sunlight, and near me lay that silent form, the red stripes of the Navajo blanket mocking the dead by their color looking so gaudy in the glare of the sunshine. Youth, hope, happiness, all changed in a second to dead, lifeless clay.

It grew very hot on that hill as the sun got overhead, for the scrub oaks were small and gave little shade. I made a back rest of my saddle, and wrote out my notes in my casebook. I saw that Dick was lying on some rocks, and moved the body more into the shade to a level place. I knew he could not feel anything in this world again, but I suppose I wanted to do something and by instinct was trying to make him look a little more comfortable.

The time certainly seemed to drag. Noon came, and I grew very thirsty. The shadows grew longer. I wondered if anything had happened to Dutch. I might have to spend the night here watching Dick. I got some sticks together so that I could light a fire to guide the boys if it grew dark. My horse neighed, and I saw him wheel and look down. Then I heard the rattle of stones, the heavy breathing of men and horses, a gruff word or two, and they gathered about the prone figure. They got to work, lashed the body to long poles, and tied the poles at one end to a saddle horse, making an Indian travois. One man led the horse, another lifted the ends of the poles over bad going, as they dragged on the ground far back of the horse. So, silently and gently these rough men carried the body to camp and laid it in the shadow of the wagon. Charlie Thompson, the captain, came in late and at once took charge while we all helped to dig a grave and bury Murphy a little way out of camp, on higher ground. We just rolled him in his blanket, put his big hat over his face, covered him with brush, and then, after piling stones so the coyotes could not get him, we went back to supper.

We all sat on our heels around the fire, cowboylike, or lounged back on our saddles or our bedrolls. The sun was almost down, and the gulches became black shadows as the night breeze came up and rustled the leaves of the scrub oak. Very faintly came the yap of the first night coyote, back to the dark hills. The horse wranglers got up stiffly and, with a "Time to get a move on, Cap," mounted and rode off. There was a clatter of stones and a thud of hoofs as the night herd moved slowly down the river to better grass and was lost in the dust and twilight, the musical tinkle of the bell growing fainter and fainter. At times the wind carried to our ears the soft murmur of the river as the water turned and twisted among the stones of the ford. It was very quiet and peaceful. The boys talked in lowered voices, with none of the usual rough jokes and banter. We were all thinking of Dick. The camp seemed dull without his happy laughter and jokes. The hardest old-timer around that fire, used as he was to sudden death by violence, was sobered by the death of this happy boy and, in his rough way, he was sorry for the little woman and baby left so helpless back there in the town. All of us kept looking at Charlie Thompson as if we expected him to say something, and at last he stood up and took off his hat.

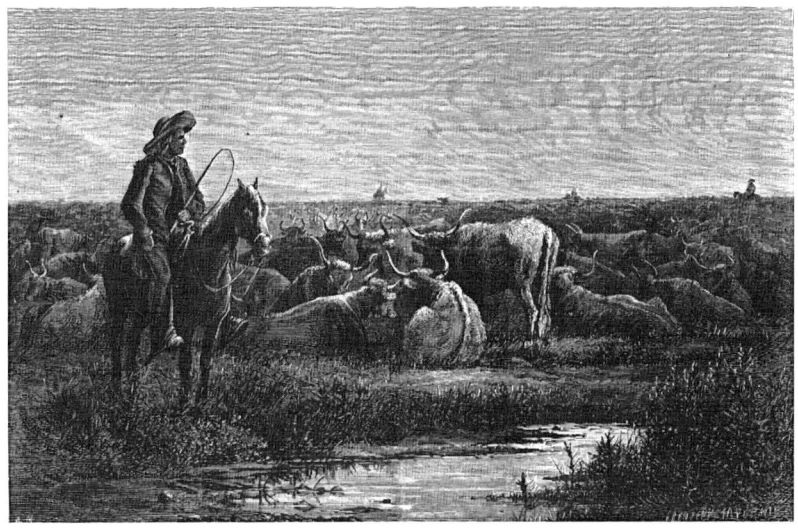

Charlie Thompson was a fine six feet of real man. His light curly hair waved in the breeze. "Boys," said Charlie, "I ain't much on the talk, but I have been milling this matter around in my head, and you all can do as you like. I ain't boss in this; it's just an idea. Now you all know that this Murphy got himself killed by riding a poor horse in a bad place. He didn't have nothing, and his wife and baby in town is dead broke, and I says to myself, let's all chip in a calf or so and start a herd. We had a good winter; we done well and won't miss it none, and it will be a living for the little widow. Now we must go slow. You see, she may be touchy-like, being beholden to us menfolk, so I think we'll send Smith up to town in the morning to break it gentle, and to tell her her man had a herd hid down the river and was calculating to surprise her a whole lot after the roundup by telling her about it. Now, Smith is the d—— est liar in Colorado, being a sailor once, and can pull this job off in great shape." Everybody said, "Sure we will, Charlie, and glad to," and we turned in. I noticed Smith took the remarks about his lying with a grin, as if at a compliment; so all was well.

Smith got away on his mission at sunup; the rest went to work. John Hills had a bad fall over a calf, and broke his collarbone, but I strapped him up, and he was riding again in a day or so.

We kept wondering how Smith was coming on. He was a curious character, not at all the ideal cowboy. He had been at sea, and told us many stories of his life; at last he had wandered up into Colorado, and by hard work had collected quite a bunch of cattle. He was a small, dark man, bowlegged, and with his old hat flapping, his red sweater, and big trousers tied by strings around his ankles, he looked funny enough. We all joked him, but he was a terror to fight, and could use a gun with the best; and, after all, he was a favorite with the boys, for he was generous and sound at heart. When he came riding in about sundown six days later, we were all glad to see him, and made him tell his story.

Smith was not what you call a beauty at his best, and on his return from his trip to town, he surely looked the worse for wear; or, as one boy expressed it, as if he had tried to stop a rockslide with his face. He was all cut up, one eye was swollen shut, and he had to eat with one side of his mouth, his lip was so badly swollen, but he grinned and took our fun as a matter of course.

When we all cleaned our tin plates off and gathered around the fire again to smoke, he opened up with his story: "Well, boys," he began, "I sure was kinder bogged down at the idea of meeting that widow and giving her your fancy lies. When I reached town and corraled my bronco, I had half a mind to have a couple of drinks at the O. K. to buck me up, but feared she'd smell liquor on me and think I was drunk, and so I just kept on to her shack, and she let me in, and I told her about her husband. Boys, I gentled it all I could, she being that small and timidlike, but she just let out a yell and cried and carried on something awful. She flung about so fierce I had to hold the baby for a spell, and I was half wild myself, what with fearing I would hold him too tight and mebby break something in him, me not savvying babies none, and fearing I'd lose my holt on him and let him fall. So when I come to tell her about the bunch of cattle and the rest of it, I was a-sweating so bad I had to open the door for air. After a time she come around fine, said she always felt her man was a born cattleman anyhow, and let on she was sure going to have some lawyer man take charge, for one never knew about these cowboys, and she, being alone, must be protected or they would sure steal all she had.

"So that went all right, and some women come along and was a-comforting her when I left. I felt like I had been wrestling with a big steer, that weak and low-minded, and I just went over to the O. K. Saloon and had a few drinks to cheer me up a bit. And since you boys left there's a new barkeep at the O. K.—a mean skunk with red hair, and he comes over to me and says, 'That story you told the Murphy widow is all bunk.' I just naturally hit him on his red head with my gun, and then things all got mussed up. How we both got back of the bar, and down fighting on a heap of broken bottles, gets me, but there we was, and when the boys pried us loose we was all blood, and whisky running off us, and my redheaded barkeep was being carried off on a board; so, not wanting no arguments or trouble on the kind of sad trip I was on, I just naturally got my horse and came a-running to camp so you all could know what I done in this widow business. And say, Charlie," he called across the fire to our captain, "I done what I could this time, but no more of them death notices and cattle lies to widows for me; you all hear me?" shaking his flappy hat over his swollen, scarred face he crowded into his bedroll. We all told him "he done fine," but only deep and harsh curses rewarded us.

We kept on combing the steers down from the hills for two weeks, and then we had the big herd all safe and sound in the valley. The roundup from east of the river brought their cattle in too, and we were busy from morning to night cutting out and branding, all in a cloud of dust fit to choke a man to death. We told the boys of the east roundup about the widow's herd we were collecting, and, fine and generous as ever, they chipped in, so we had quite a bunch of cattle for the little woman. It was mostly she-stock, so the increase would count up, and Captain Thompson went to Denver and had her brand recorded in the regular way, that she might have no trouble. The lawyer engaged to protect her interests put in an appearance in town, and when he heard our story, insisted that he meant "to write the little fool the real truth," but the boys made him promise not to, for it was such a good joke on them to be suspected of stealing from the widow, that it was a shame to spoil the joke. They really did have many a laugh over it, and it was a byword ever after to call out, "Say, you're stealing from the widow." Cowboy humor is curious at times.

When I got back to town Mrs. Murphy was dressed in black, and looked very small and forlorn; she was going home to Carolina, Mother White having given her the money. The next morning we turned out to see her off, a four-days' ride to the railroad. As the stage rocked and rolled away, a small handkerchief fluttered out of the window, and we saw the mother and baby for a moment. Then a cloud of dust hid everything.

The boys kept the widow's herd up for some years, and then sold out at top prices and sent the money to a trust company in the South. Mrs. Murphy wrote a note to Charlie Thompson saying "she was well provided for, all due to the knowledge and skill of her lamented husband who, if he had lived, would have been a Cattle King."

Charlie laughed and said, "Well, it's a good thing she never caught on."

Chapter 5
My Tenderfoot

I had been expecting my tenderfoot for several days. An old college friend had written to me that he had a young fellow among his patients who was just recovering from an attack of typhoid fever, and whose people were anxious about him. He was still nervous and run down, needing a change from New York and its noises; therefore, he had advised this young man, who was just out of college, to go out West to Colorado and rough it for a time. My friend knew I would look after his patient if he came to me; so for several days I watched the stage come in, and got into the habit of referring to "my tenderfoot."

At last the day arrived. We were all out in front of the only store awaiting the arrival of our stage. It was the one event of the day, for it was our only link with the outside world and the news. The railroad was just one hundred fifty miles away, over a road that, in places, was but little more than a trail; a road that was, in different seasons, deep in alkali dust, or hub deep in sticky mud, and when the snow was deep, almost impassable; a road that had no bridges, only fords that in flood filled the coach with muddy water and soaked the passengers and mail sacks with impartial disregard of consequences; a road that was full of rocks and holes and terrible hills. Consequently, a stage in those old days was tossed and bumped along until every bolt and brace in its structure was strained to the limit.

You started out gaily enough from the railroad in a big Concord coach with six horses, all excited to be able to ride in a coach, away out West in the keen air, where one saw antelope and deer, and men wearing guns and wide hats. After seventy-five miles you drew up at a small dirty cabin, wherein you ate a greasy mess of pork and beans and soggy bread; you lay on the dirt floor all night and were very cold; and in the morning, upon washing your face in a dirty basin, you found the water like ice and the roller towel quite black. It was just dawn, and the coffee you had for breakfast tasted like bitter mud. You ate more greasy pork, and then, no coach! But in its place was the "jerky," a six-seated buckboard piled with boxes and mail sacks and no place to put your legs. Hour after hour you bumped among the boxes. The sun seemed to burn your clothes; the dust choked and smothered you; and the road seemed endless. Then came another night on a hard dirt floor, with the air very cold, for you were now up eight thousand feet. You could not sleep, and with horror you found things crawling over you and biting you. Then another day, and you found the road getting worse every foot; and soon, after being rocked and twisted, tired and stiff, nearly a wreck, you crawled out at our place, which was the end of the road.

It was wonderful to see the change that road produced on innocent and unfortunate travelers. They would leave the comfortable train all dolled up with new things, everything shiny and bright, beautiful Stetson hats, shiny rifles, spotless belts and leggings, with saddles, blankets, and luggage enough for a year at least. These same tenderfeet arrived with burnt faces and bruised bodies, and painfully and stiffly crawled out

My Tenderfoot

from their seats of torture among hard boxes and mail sacks, all covered with dust and grime, so shaky they could hardly stand. In faint and husky voices they asked for the hotel, amid a circle of grinning cowpunchers, wild with delight at the unusual spectacle of these city dudes being "shaken down" in the wilderness.

So, it was with some curiosity that I watched the stage come lumbering up to the store that hot July afternoon and saw a slim youth sitting slumped down in a back seat, almost too tired to move. But as he looked up, and I gave my name, he greeted me with a feeble smile. Covered with white dust, burned a brick red, and barely able to stand, he looked a wreck. So, shouldering his bag, I soon had him in bed in my cabin. The next morning, after his shave and breakfast, I had a chance to size him up. He was about twenty years of age, fresh from New York and Columbia, still weak from typhoid, very much a gentleman, quiet and modest. He was a likable young fellow, and I took a fancy to him at once.

I very soon arranged a program for him to follow. Of course he was wild to shoot at the big game that was so easily hunted in those days. At first I feared to let him roam around alone, for he was a rank tenderfoot, as green as grass, and knew nothing of the country or about handling weapons. I was a bit worried as to how the cowboys would treat this rare specimen from the city, and was at first a little dubious about his meeting the boys in the general store or the saloon. However, I was doing an injustice to the cowpunchers, for they size up a man very quickly, and are always ready to be fair. This tenderfoot of mine had a natural modesty, a charm of manner, and such an instinctive admiration for men who did things and were simple and true, that, to my surprise, he became a prime favorite overnight, and could be seen at any time hobnobbing with some of our most noted bad men, and laughing at their jokes. They entered with great interest into his outfit, helped him buy a gentle pony, saddle, bridle, and rope. In a short time they had taught him the way to ride, how to care for his horse, and many of the details of their work.

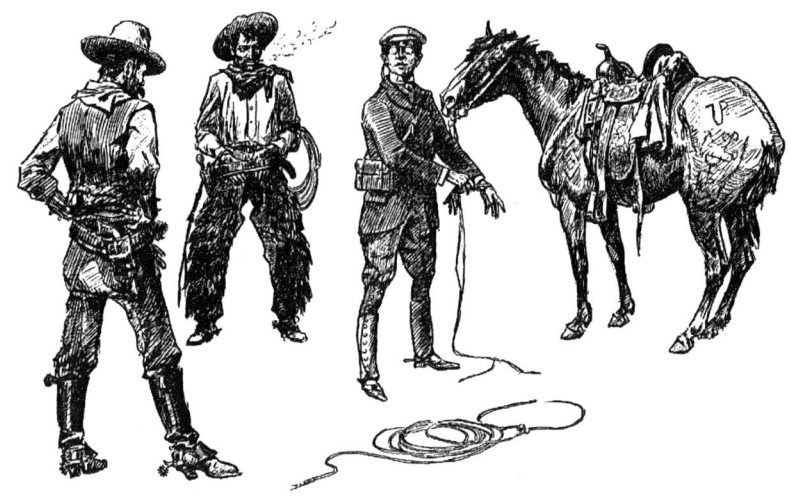

It was natural that the boy should fall in love with the life, for our little cow town, so far away from the crowded centers in the East, had a charm, in spite of the rough and lawless conditions. We were in a little valley about a mile above the sea level, where the air was very dry and clear, and there were just a few cabins on both sides of our only street. By these cabins ran a river some one hundred yards across—a clear mountain stream fed by the snows of the main range. It was full of trout, while groves of cottonwoods and pine trees lined the banks, and little meadows dotted with wild flowers made the scenes like some parks seen in the East. The surroundings were like a New England village, with trees, green grass, and water. To the north towered the high, snow-covered peaks of the main range of the Rocky Mountains, sheer spires of dazzling white snow against the deep blue sky. Below them lay the dense deep green of the forests of spruce and pines. Here and there a brook, alive with native trout, came running down from the mountains through little parks where there were elk, deer, and the big silvertip bear. No wonder the boy liked it and wrote glowing letters to his family.

My Tenderfoot

There was an old hunter named Ned Smith, who, for a small fee, took my boy in charge; and great was the excitement when they came back with the heads of elk and deer, and there was mounting of heads and skins, especially of a mountain lion they had come upon in a tree and shot. Now that my tenderfoot was growing stronger every day and feeling more at home, he suggested one day that he take a little trip down the river to see something of the roundups, branding, and horse breaking going on there. I had no anxiety over his safety. I gave him a letter to the foreman of the O. T. I., down about thirty-five miles, and, as the boy did not drink or gamble, but was a quiet and modest lad, I felt he was safe enough. He would have been but for that "half sister of fate," called "Chance." There was not more than one possibility in a thousand that any trouble could come to him. And yet the one in a thousand did happen, because of a rare combination of circumstances.

Of course, we were living in rather a lawless community where might meant right—more or less—and any established order of things came later. That summer the cattle thieves became so active all over the country—even in the summer ranges up in the mountains—that the cattlemen determined to put them down. They called on a detective agency in Denver, which sent out young fellows disguised as cowboys, who rode the range and spotted rustlers whom they reported to the agency. Of course, the rustlers knew this, and were looking for these detectives. They had shot one or two who did not play their part well enough. Consequently, all the cattle thieves were jumpy, suspicious, and ready at any time or place to shoot it out at the drop of a hat.

Now, there was a man called "Reddy" who, for some months, rode for a ranch up the river near us, and we all knew him to be a bad actor in ordinary times. When he was drunk he was a devil. It was rumored that he had killed a man in Wyoming, and that he really was a cattle thief and worked at riding only to cover up his tracks. At any rate, the ranch people above our place let him out in the spring, and he was now working down the river near where my tenderfoot was intending to visit.

But the last idea in my head at that time was to connect my tenderfoot—such a mild, innocent youth—with such a drunken man-killer as Reddy.

I had almost forgotten my tenderfoot, for I expected him to be gone a week at least, when, after three days, a man rode in to have me treat his hand, which he had cut in a barbwire fence. He lived only a few miles away, but I asked him, as usual, what the news was and how he was getting on. He said a range rider from down the river who had gone by his place just before he left, had told him that somebody had shot and killed Reddy down in Mex Joe's near the breaking corral.

I heard nothing more until noon the next day, when I saw two riders coming to my place. They were Black, head boss of the T. O. B., and my tenderfoot. As they drew up at my cabin I thought the boy looked sick, and when he got off I had to help him to stand. I asked him if he felt sick, and he said, "No, only tired," and passed into the cabin. Later I put him into bed, and he said, "I can't talk, Doctor, please give me something to make me sleep." I gave him a big dose of bromide.

When I went out and asked Black what had happened to the boy, Black said, "Well, Doc, I can't tell you much. You see, we boys is camped at the mouth of Yellow Creek, and this kid spent the night with us, and rode on down the river to see some branding at the breaking corral. The next night, as we was hitting the blankets about nine o'clock, in comes Charlie Walker from the night herd, bringing this kid, plumb lost, and his horse trailing him to our place. All night this kid kept walking up and back by the fire, would eat nothing, and seemed to be just awfully worried about something. He didn't say anything and, of course, Doc, the boys just pretended not to notice nothing strange, as it was his own business. In the morning he was all of a jump to be going on his way. I knew he was dead sure to be lost, him being kind of nutty that way, and I just saddled up and said I had to come to town to get some tobacco, as I was all out. Of course I had tobacco aplenty, but I felt I must ride along to guard him a bit, and lied about the tobacco so he would suspicion nothing. So here we are, and I don't know

My Tenderfoot

what's a-biting the kid." And off rode Black to have a drink or so, and then go back to camp.

It took several days to get the story out of my tenderfoot, but in any case the whole country knew it by that time. I saw the judge, Mex Joe, and some of the boys working at the corral at different times, and they all said the story was as the Tenderfoot told it to me.

My tenderfoot told his tale very simply, but was evidently overcome by the horror of it.

After leaving our place that morning when he started on his trip, he had ridden for miles through the park country where the trail wound by the riverbank. This was a well-marked trail, first made by deer and elk, and then used by the cattlemen as they drove their herds up and down the river. He stopped at a pool and had lunch while his horse grazed on the thick grass; he was thrilled to see big trout jumping in the river and resolved to go fishing at the first opportunity. That afternoon he came on a summer camp where three or four cowboys were stationed to turn their cattle up to the higher pastures along Yellow Creek, that ran into the main river at this point. He knew two of the men, and they made much of the boy, turned his horse into the night herd, helped him with his bedroll, and showed him the mess wagon. Then he sat with them around the fire and heard their yarns about Indians and shooting scrapes. He was enchanted with the life, and when they saddled his horse in the morning and rode a bit of the trail with him on his way, and then with a "So long, Kid," rode off on their business, he felt he was having a glorious time. Mile after mile he rode along, never seeing a human being.

The air was so clear and bracing, and the sunlight was so bright that he could see the snow fields on the Great Divide, and every detail of their valleys and peaks, far up in the blue fifty miles away, as if you could walk to them in an hour. He thought of his family in their brownstone house on Fifth Avenue; his gray-haired father, so kind and dignified; everything in the house running like clockwork; and of his mother, anxious over him, and proud of his college standing. How shocked they would be in their conventional and correct life, to hear his stories of the wild animals and rough men! How his college friends would envy him when the big deer head and mountain lion skins were shown them in his study. He was awakened from these daydreams when, riding up on a hill, he saw below him a mile or so on, a corral by the river. The faint breeze carried to him the smell of burnt hair, the bawling of the calves, and the harsh shouts of men. In the corral he saw smoke coming from a small fire, and saw men bending over it, others on horseback riding around the corral, swinging their ropes over their heads and roping calves that galloped this way and that in frantic fear, to avoid the big loop's descending over their heads.

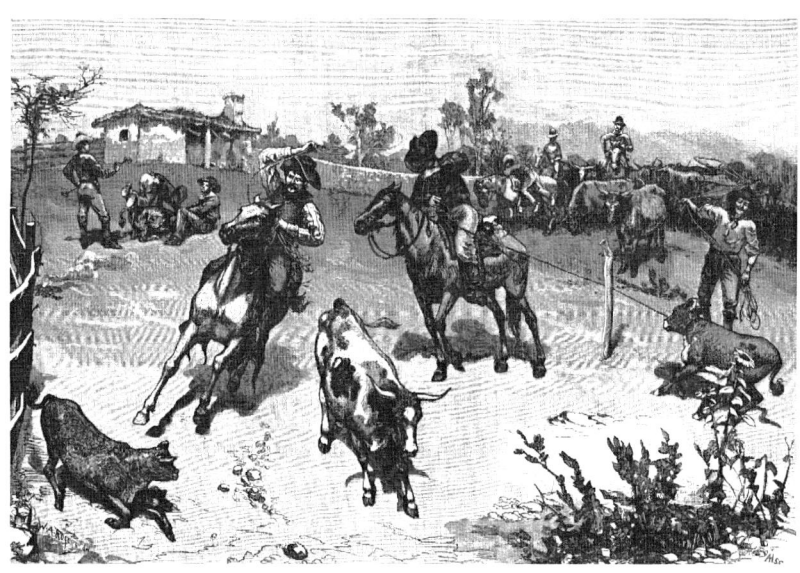

So this was the place where he would see the cattle business! Feeling the letter in his pocket, which he was to deliver to Kelly, he rode eagerly forward to find him. As he got nearer he saw several cabins in a row, and a board building like a general store. The first cabin he came to was a low one, made of upright poles and mud; he saw the door was half open, and he heard voices. A horse stood outside by the door, the reins on the ground, patiently waiting for his owner, as only a bronco can. He tied his horse to a tree, leaving his rifle in its case. This was the only weapon he had, for I had advised him not to bother with a revolver. He walked over to the cabin, and pushing the door open, he looked inside. It was dark after the bright sunshine outside, but gradually he made out a long table, several rough chairs, and at one end a rude kind of bar made of planks, with a few bottles in a row on a shelf; thousands of flies hummed as they surged back and forth in a dense swarm near the dirty canvas ceiling. A Mexican leaned over the bar. He was an evil-looking brute, short and dark, with a most villainous face, an earring in one ear, and a bright red handkerchief tied around his head of jet-black hair. He was leaning over the bar and talking in a low voice, in a servile, coaxing way, to a man who lounged over the bar opposite him. This man was of a powerful build, with a dark, flushed, sunburnt face. His big hat was tilted back, and a shock of fiery hair stood up all over his head, against the broad brim. He wore a flannel shirt and chaps, and from each hip hung a big revolver on the low-slung belt. He wore large Mexican spurs on his boots and, as he moved, they tinkled like bells. He was very drunk, and staggered a bit when he moved. He was evidently in a rage, for his voice was almost a shout as he cursed and raved his threats at the Mexican, who was evidently trying to smooth the matter over. He was saying, "I tell you, Mex, I heard yesterday that a d—— detective agency in Denver is sending out a lot of skunk spies dressed up like tenderfeet, as if they knew nothing, and they're smelling around to spy on us. I'll show 'em good and plenty if I find 'em." At this point my tenderfoot meant to draw back, but as they both saw him, he felt he would better go in. Addressing the Mexican, he asked where he could find Jim Kelly, as he had a letter to him.

Now Kelly, unfortunately, had been most active in running down cattle and horse thieves, and was away on a trip at the time. The Mexican answered briefly, "He's away now." All this time, the big man called Reddy, was regarding my tenderfoot intensely, taking in his clothes and his face with an insolent stare that made the boy very nervous. His manner probably conveyed to Reddy's muddled brain a consciousness of guilt. The name of Kelly seemed to arouse a sudden devil in Reddy for, to the surprise and horror of the boy, he suddenly strode forward, seized the boy by his neck, forced him back against the wall of the cabin, half choking him, drew a gun, and forcing the end of the barrel into his stomach, shouted, "I know you, you d—— detective, a-monkeying around and spying on us; I'll just kill you, you son of a ——, right now." The Mex called, "Oh, go easy, Red, he's only a kid!" Reddy, glancing over his shoulders, shouted, "You shut your black mouth, you dirty Mex."

My tenderfoot, paralyzed with fear, said he knew nothing about detectives, mentioned my name, and begged the man to read the letter he had for Kelly. But it was of no use, for Reddy was wild and only pushed him harder and shook him like a rat. At this moment a yell was heard from the corral. "Oh, Reddy, come here. Can't read this brand." With an oath Reddy flung the boy aside; half conscious the boy fell across a chair and lay there panting. Reddy paused in the doorway, and with an oath growled out, "You try to skin out and I'll shoot you in the open," and was gone. As my tenderfoot lay gasping on the chair, he heard the clatter of hoofs as Reddy tore off for the corral. Half sick from terror, he turned desperately to Joe, the Mexican barkeeper, saying, "For God's sake hide me or he will come back and murder me!" The next instant Joe vaulted over the bar, shoved a big revolver into his hand, saying, in a hoarse whisper, "Hurry, Kid! Get behind the door and shoot him as he comes in or you are a dead one. I know Reddy!"

The Mexican crawled out through a loose place in the wall, and was gone. Shaking with fear, as if in some horrid dream, my tenderfoot sprang back of the half-open door and crouched, in a panic of fear. He heard the clatter of a galloping horse and, looking through a crack back of the door, saw Reddy riding at a furious pace toward the cabin. There was a sliding rattle of gravel, some dust blown into the doorway, and he could see Reddy spring from the saddle with his revolver in his hand. The light was shut out as the big body swayed through the doorway, the brim of a big hat came out from the edge of the door, followed by a face with a sunburnt space below the ear. As Reddy called out "Where is that —— detective?" tremblingly the tenderfoot pushed the gun he held in both hands within an inch of that dark patch below the ear and fired. The shot sounded like a cannon. His hands jerked with the recoil, and a dense cloud of powder smoke hid everything for a moment. There was an instant of silence, broken only by the buzzing of thousands of flies, like the waves of the sea, as they surged overhead. He could hear a curious scratching, and peering fearfully around the edge of the door, saw two hands grasping the rough post of the doorway in a futile effort to hold on. Then came a thud as the relaxed body fell on the dirt floor, a silvery tinkle like a bell as a spur on a trembling foot quivered for an instant and then grew still. The big hat covered the head and neck as the body fell, face down, and from under the brim a dark pool was spreading, and the buzzing flies were gathering, while overhead the swarm, startled by the shot, flew back and forth like a black cloud, and there was a buzzing sound like the thunder of a distant surf beating on the shore.

 My boy flung himself across the bar, half fainting. He wanted to escape somewhere, away from that awful cabin with its smell of burnt powder and blood, but could not face that door with that form sprawled across the threshold. His breath came in gasps, and the humming of the multitude of flies drove him nearly crazy. He gave a jump as a hand grasped his wrist, and a voice said, "Drink this." A glass was put to his lips, and chokingly he gulped down the fiery whisky. The Mexican bent over him, saying, "Come, Kid, hurry up. We must see the justice!" He passively allowed the Mexican to lead him. It was all like a nightmare; he could not believe it was real. With averted eyes he stepped over the body of Reddy, lying so strangely quiet and still. Then he was blinking in the bright sunlight outside.

Hurriedly he was led by the Mexican to a cabin where a sign on the door read, "Justice of the Peace." As if in a dream he remembered entering the cabin. At a table in the middle of the room sat a tall old man with a white beard. He sat tilted back, his feet on the table, his thumbs in the armholes of a very dirty vest. A glass of whisky stood on the table, and by its side a pair of the biggest revolvers the boy had ever seen. Without moving a muscle of his lined old face, this individual solemnly stared at the two visitors and, without a word, he spat with wonderful skill into an old box filled with sand beside him. The Mexican grew nervous and kept shifting his feet in a restless way, looking this way and that with his black eyes, as if anxious to escape. At last he blurted out, "Your Honor, Reddy was fitting to kill this kid. I heard him, and the kid just naturally shot him."

In a deep slow drawl the justice asked the Mexican, "Is Reddy dead?"

"Yes, sir, deader 'n hell."

"Come here," said the justice. As my tenderfoot stood in front of him, he pointed a long finger at him, saying, "Young man, you get on your horse, and you ride north and don't stop for nothing until you reach your friends." And that was all.

My tenderfoot was amazed and relieved, and stammered some thanks, only to be cut short by the justice's saying, "Two bucks for the court fee." Gladly the boy handed over the two dollars, and in a backward glance through the doorway, he saw the justice sitting in the same position, his feet on the table, tilted back in his chair, and hitting the box with tobacco juice with unmoved skill. Still in a dream my tenderfoot mounted his horse, pressed five dollars into Joe's hand, and was away. Completely lost, he reached the camp in the dark. The old-time cowboy was rather a wise man, it is true, but these men never asked him a question. They gave him a bed, took care of his horse, and saw him off in the morning with a "So long." A gentleman had nothing to teach these cowboys of the open range in tact and consideration.

My Tenderfoot

I had my tenderfoot patched up in a few days, and although he seemed to play rather a sorry part in his little drama, and even appeared to be a near coward, I do not think he was at all lacking in courage. The circumstances were peculiar; he was strange to the country and weakened by an illness; and the surprise and fear of the unusual tested him beyond his strength. It was no wonder that he was shocked and nervous from his trying experience.

As I saw my tenderfoot off on the stage for his long journey to New York and his family, I was much touched by his gratitude and thanks for the little service I had done for him. In good time I had also a letter of appreciation from his father, and the innocent gentleman—bless his simple heart—wanted to know if any "legal action was likely to ensue from the unfortunate occasion that had so shocked and distressed his son." Needless to say, there was no legal question, and the sentiment in our community can be briefly and somewhat coarsely expressed in the words of our esteemed and cheerful barkeeper at the I. X. L. Saloon, who, hearing of the distress shown by my tenderfoot at his tragic encounter, said, "Well, Doc, what's biting the kid? He killed Reddy, didn't he? Then, what in hell is he kicking about?"

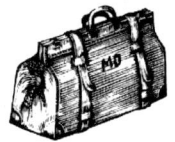

Chapter 6
A Tenderfoot Sheriff

Silver Cup lay half asleep, while a long line of broncos, saddled and bridled, were tied to the hitch rails in front of the saloons and stores. It was horsefly season, and the big flies buzzed and crawled over the broncos that stood switching their tails and stamping the dust. At last a big horsefly reached a secure position under a bronco at the end of the line, where ordinary kicking failed to dislodge him. There was a shrill scream as, half frantic with the sting, the poor brute commenced to buck and kick. Down the line the panic ran like a prairie fire, and one after another all the broncos began rearing and kicking. The hitch rail bent and creaked under the strain. A citizen, shirt-sleeved and hatless, burst forth from the swing door of a saloon and, much excited, ran up and down the boardwalk in front of the pitching and kicking horses. His language exceeded any ordinary cursing as a river does a brook. Even the broncos were appalled, and soon relapsed into their ordinary bored attitudes. The citizen, red and breathless from the strain, paused for a moment at the saloon door to hurl a parting threat full of hell-fire at the now subdued broncos, then went in to his poker game again.

As the sun got lower, and the gulches turned a purple tint, the town woke up a bit. Miners were coming in from their claims, mud covered and weary as they tramped along, some with pack on back, some on horseback, the drills tied to their saddles clinking as they trotted past. Then the long trains of burros, each with its load of ore on packsaddle, went slowly past, their little hoofs stirring up a yellow cloud of dust. Dimly seen at the end of the line, a man rode a bronco, carelessly sitting on his horse, lounging in the saddle with one leg over the horse as if weary with the slow pace; but with any straying of his small charges in front, he at once became violent and profane, throwing rocks and casting horrible insults at the unfortunate offenders. Big ore wagons, their hind wheels locked, went sliding down the last pitch of the road into camp, bumping and rumbling over rocks, the six mules handled with the skill that only an old-time mule skinner possessed.

A crowd collected on the boardwalk outside the general store and post office. The main event of the day—the arrival of the mail coach—was waited for with impatience. Finally a small boy cried in a shrill voice, "There she is!" and down the valley along the main road, winding in and out among the hills below, there rose a cloud of dust; soon the lead team came around a corner at a gallop and then the big Concord coach, rocking like a ship at sea, came into sight. The crowd cheered. The coach, with rattle of doubletrees, whining of brakes, and pounding of six horses, made a wide circle, lead and swing teams galloping. The coach was brought to a stop at the exact spot chosen, missing the walk by an inch. The passengers scrambled out through the doors and down from the top, weary, stiff, and dust covered. Mail sacks were thrown from the boot.

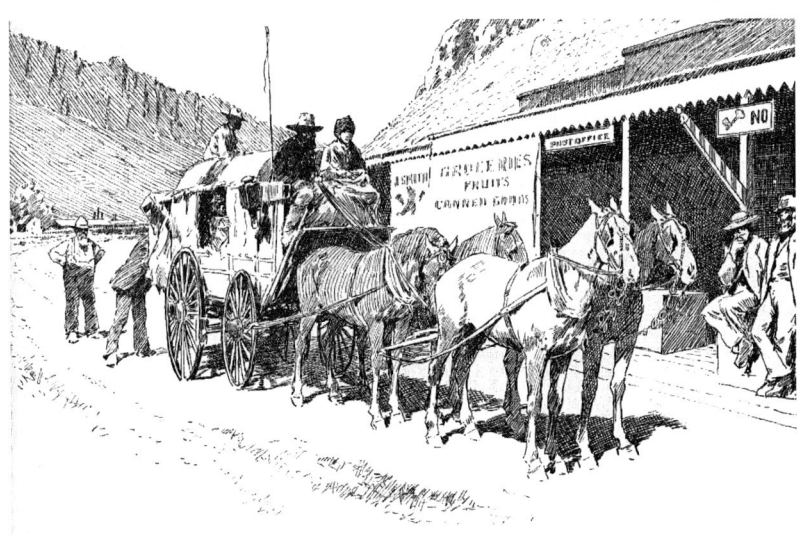

From his seat beside the driver, the express messenger handed down his ironbound treasure chest to a tall dark man with a big handkerchief around his neck, and a pair of hard, keen eyes in his head. He cast a swift look over the crowd as if seeking trouble, and crashed the chest down on the counter with a look of relief. Safe this trip, anyhow, he no doubt felt. Armed with Winchester and revolver, the messenger, in a leisurely fashion, descended with the dignity befitting his dangerous duty and followed his precious box into the post office.

The last man to descend was slow and careful, and it was seen that he had a limp, was pale of face, thin, and looked ill. He coughed painfully as he dragged his bag along the walk; evidently the dust on the long ride had irritated his lungs, or, as some suspected, he was a "lunger." He looked about twenty-five, and "tenderfoot" was stamped all over him. Almost unnoticed, he asked a passerby where he could find a boardinghouse, and was directed to Mother White's place. He breathlessly thanked the man and was seen to stagger into the house of Mother White. No doubt the altitude was hard on him, for the air is thin at nine thousand feet. No one saw him for some weeks. The doctor reported him as getting better, for the air was curing him, he said. Finally the sick tenderfoot began to stir about a little, and gradually he became known to most of the people about, a shy, modest sort of man, never taking a drink, or gambling, for, he said, it was bad for his health. He seemed to have enough money for his wants, was always polite, and, as Mrs. White said, was a "regular gentleman."

Strange things used to happen in the old days in mining camps. Strange people blew into camp—from bishops to blacklegs—but of all the queer people, this quiet youth gave us a new twist. As I have said, no one noticed him much. He was a "lunger," taking the air on our high mountains to cure him. Then, as the summer wore on, and he was so much better, he took long walks alone, and it was noticed that he always selected some quiet gulch from which revolver shots were later heard. No one paid any attention to this; if the tenderfoot wanted to shoot at a mark, let him go to it. Finally old man Tracy, a bum who was always sticking his nose into everything, declared he was "a-going to see what this tenderfoot was a-shooting at up them gulches," so he trailed the stranger up a gulch and watched him.

When Tracy returned from his spying he was so surprised and breathless that it took three whiskies to fit him to talk, and then he gave out a yarn that no one believed. He said that he hid behind a rock and saw this tenderfoot do some fancy shooting that made his eyes fairly start out of his head. "Why, boys," he exclaimed, "that bird threw up bottles, shot and broke 'em in the air."

The boys gave him the horselaugh. "You damned old fool," they roared, "you was drunk and dreamt it." Now the idea of any Eastern tenderfoot coming into the West and being a real gunman was too ridiculous to entertain for a moment and, as Andy McKay said, "That white-livered little lame duck can't shoot nothing." It was difficult to believe. That this delicate youth, still wearing a derby hat and "store" clothes, precise in speech, and never taking a drink, could have even a speaking knowledge of a Colt revolver, was a joke.

There was much argument over the story old man Tracy gave out, and to settle the question it was decided to see this tenderfoot, who called himself Smith, and ask him about his shooting. So a number of the old-timers, led by Kelly, barkeeper and owner of the best saloon in town, walked over to Mrs. White's place and called on Mr. Smith. Mr. Smith appeared rather anxious, wondering, no doubt, what sinister motive was in the air to inspire such a call. However, being assured that the visit was a friendly one, he became most cordial and, when told of old man Tracy's spying, was much amused. "Now, gentlemen," said Mr. Smith, "I will tell you all about myself. There is no mystery about my life. Some of you may have seen my name on circus posters down East. I am called the wonder shot of the world. I am a circus man, born in winter quarters in Connecticut. My family are well-known circus people, called the Le Clair family. Father is a bareback rider, and Mother does some slack-wire and trapeze work. As a kid I fell from a "trap" and broke my hip. That put me out of the regular line, as I had a limp. Finding I had a sort of natural ability at throwing stones and hitting things, Father taught me to use a revolver. I kept hard at it day after day, and finally I was so good that at nineteen I had an act all to myself, shooting glass balls thrown in the air—not in the big tent, but outside in a side show. Then I did the same act on horseback. I had a kind of gift that way, I suppose. I used both rifle and revolver, but the revolver act took the people more. Anyhow, I was making good money with the circus when I took consumption and had to quit. I was told to go to Colorado, and came up here in the mountains. I am so much better now that I go out every day to some quiet spot to shoot and stay in practice so I can keep my hand in and be able to go back to the circus when I am well."

Smith was so quiet and modest that he quite won over his visiting committee, and they returned to the saloon to report. Many were still very doubtful, and to cut the matter short and test this circus man's skill, it was unanimously voted that a real test of his shooting was the only fair method to settle the question. And to spare his feeling and not make a holy show of him by asking him to display his skill alone, with the tact and consideration often shown by frontiersmen, they felt it was best to have a sort of contest. There were plenty of wonderful revolver shots in town, one called "Oregon Bill" being the best. Oregon Bill was a gambler of the higher type, who always dressed and acted quite the gentleman. Quiet and polite, he was known by all to be fair and honest. No one was more esteemed as a citizen and good fellow. It was difficult to induce him to show his skill, but one bit of shooting I saw myself. He threw an empty tomato can into the road in front of Bill's horse, and Bill, riding at a lope, would shoot his revolver at the can so that every bullet would just clip the top side of the can and keep it rolling along the road until it was nicked so badly that it could not roll any more. He never seemed to take any aim—just threw his gun down as if snapping a whip. It looked easy, but try it, mounted on a restless horse, and see! We had others that could hit a potato thrown into the air, once in two or three times, so there were plenty of gunmen about to choose from, and the betting on the contest assumed a stage as acute as a horse race.

A Tenderfoot Sheriff

The next morning a queer procession was seen proceeding up a small canyon near town: some were on horseback, some on foot; all were joking and making fun out of it. In the midst, riding with a quiet smile on his pale face, came the circus man, Smith. Arriving at a little level space, we found sacks of potatoes and tin cans had been dumped down to serve as targets, as all scorned the usual fixed-paper targets with rings and black bull's-eye. The men crowded around Smith to see his revolvers, and well they might, for they had never before gazed upon a more gorgeous pair of firearms. They were the regular big forty-five Colts of the day, only in these of Smith's, art had exceeded itself in making them "a thing of beauty and a joy forever." They were intended to dazzle and astound a circus crowd. The handles were of mother-of-pearl. The barrels, covered with gold inlay in wavy designs and patterns of flowers and vines sparkled and flashed in the sunlight. As a work of art, they excited much admiration, but one old-timer was heard to exclaim in disgust, "Them guns is too damn phony for real business."

The canyon opened out into a little park covered with grass, and the trial of skill commenced by a number of the best shots setting up potatoes or tin cans at about one hundred feet. Then Oregon Bill came forward on his horse and "rolled a can." He did some splendid shooting, but the ground was rough, and the can would not roll along as on a road, so Bill dismounted, and a friend of his tossed potatoes into the air. It was fine shooting, and he hit one out of three or four.

Then the event of the day, the test of the circus man, took place. That modest individual walked out slowly in front of the crowd and quite calmly asked one of the bystanders to throw for him. A few potatoes were offered, but with a smile were declined and, to the astonishment of the entire party, Smith took from his pocket a couple of walnuts. Going up to the man who was to throw, Smith asked him to "throw these walnuts up in the air about twenty feet when I give the word." Now a walnut is almost impossible to hit with a rifle or a revolver, and the curious crowd in the background were betting ten to one against him. But nothing daunted, the quiet Smith, with a look of careless confidence on his thin features, stood back some twenty feet and gave the word "Throw!" Both walnuts mounted in the air, made graceful curves, each in its own orbit, and at the top of the curve were, for a split second, almost at rest before falling. At this fraction of time, when they seemed like black specks overhead, Smith's guns both roared out. The walnuts, smashed to small fragments, drifted off on the breeze. The spectators, looking up with open mouths, for a moment stood silent with surprise, and then gathered about Smith and

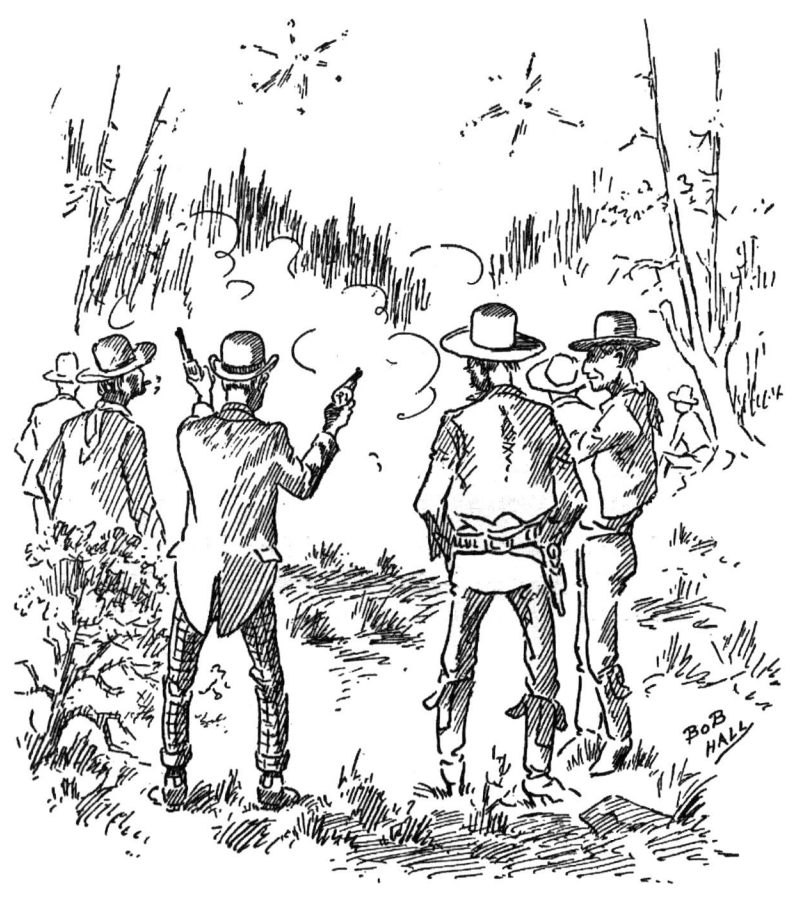

yelled, slapped him on the back, and behaved generally like crazy men. The old-timers were good sports, and the first one to shake Smith by the hand and congratulate him was Oregon Bill. Smith took his triumph and honors with becoming modesty. After all, a circus man was used to it, and no doubt Smith considered the audience a small one after his work before a big crowd at the circus.

There was some more shooting, and Smith did a few tricks that delighted the boys, such as shooting at an object behind him while he looked in a small looking glass, and riding a horse in a circle while shooting at a bottle in the middle with both guns at once. At any rate everyone was happy, even the losers. When paying up their bets, many declared it was worth the money to see such shooting. Smith's fame spread far and wide, but he took it all with a New Englander's lack of emotion, refused to show off again, and returned to his quiet pursuit of health.

About a week after this shooting contest, the sheriff of the town, Bob Mullen, became very ill. Bob was a popular character, a large hearty man in the sixties — an old-timer who was ready to gamble and drink at any time of night or day. But the "tanglefoot" was getting him, as all could see; and when the boys carried him up to his room one night, and he tearfully implored them to kill the big red spiders that "was a-covering him," many old friends shook their heads sadly, and felt that old Bob was on his last trail. And so it proved, for Bob "went over the range" that night.

There was considerable discussion as to who should be the next sheriff, the Democrats almost coming to a gun fight with the Republicans over the matter. The question seemed at a deadlock when, most of the gentlemen being weary and very drunk, one bright spirit suggested electing Smith, for, as he justly remarked, "He can shoot hell out of any damned sheriff in these mountains." The idea was hailed as a novelty; anything went in those days. A camp settled its own business. Without any more formality, Smith was then and there given the position of sheriff of Silver Cup. When informed of the compliment conferred upon him, Smith wished to refuse, explaining that he was new to the ways of the West and did not feel capable of filling the post to their satisfaction. But he was overruled, and told to "shut up." A large silver star was pinned to his coat and, in rather a dazed condition, he received the congratulations of his friends.

Now Smith, although from the East, had seen something of the rough type of men in his day and had, in fact, been in the midst of a number of circus fights when the toughs of a village made attacks on the circus people, so that he had nerve enough. But the one weak point in his experience was his ignorance of the ways of the Western men. It was a curious code they had, and rather a confusing one to a tenderfoot. If you shot a man without any warning, it was murder, and you were promptly hanged by the vigilance committee. If you shot a man who was about to shoot you, it was only a killing on the square, and nothing was done. Also the advice he got from his friends was not calculated to give him much judgment in a showdown. He was instructed to do all he could to avoid trouble but, as an old-timer informed him, "When there is real trouble, son, you turn loose both your fancy guns and shoot to kill." I fear Smith took this advice in a literal sense and did not realize the danger of overzealous action.

Like many circus people of his time, Smith was brought up very strictly; no dissipation of any kind was allowed and, strange to say, old circus families were most religious and conventional. Religion was a real force in their lives, and Smith, in the midst of all the gambling and drinking of the West, led a life apart and was unconsciously a puritan in spite of his occupation. No doubt his position as sheriff caused him many anxious moments. His sense of duty and his religious training conflicted with the reckless disregard for life and morals seen in a mining camp, so that, fearing to fall short of his duty, he was likely to overcome his fears by acting too hastily.

One day when the mail arrived, Smith got a letter which he read in the post office, and people noticed that he seemed troubled by the contents. However, he put the letter in his pocket and went over to see his friend Judge Jackson. Smith was a long time with the judge—probably asking his advice about his duties—but neither Smith nor the judge ever told what was said.

I saw this fateful letter some time later, and made a copy, for it was a queer specimen of the legal code of the day.

>Black Mesa, Colorado,
>July, 1884
>
>Sheriff's Office:
>Sir:
>
>As you is sheriff of Silver Cup, keep a looking for two outlaws, called Arizona Bill and Frenchy. They is dressed in buckskin, and is sure wild ones, came a roaring into our place drunk, and a shooting. Hit Tom Hank's boy, and pulled their freight before I could get action. They was a hedded your way when last seen.
>
>Respectfully,
>Hank Baxter,
>Sheriff.

The next morning about eleven o'clock two men rode down the almost deserted street of Silver Cup, turned their horses and, drawing up in front of Kelly's Saloon, dismounted. They tied their horses to the hitch rail in front and went into the saloon. No one around took much notice. It was sure, however, that these men were about thirty years of age, were tanned as dark as Indians, and wore full beards and long hair that hung to their shoulders. They were dressed in fringed buckskin shirts, ragged and torn from long use; they wore chaps, and big spurs on high-heeled boots. Each man had a rifle slung from his saddle, and Colt revolvers hung from his belt. Their horses were fine, spirited animals with some thoroughbred in them; their saddles and bridles were very fine, ornamented with silver. It was remarked that these men rode with the skill of born cowboys as their horses pranced and shied at the strange sights of the town. Fifty years ago it was nothing unusual to see men clothed and armed as these were coming into a mining camp. Although the fringed buckskin shirts were a bit unusual, old hunters still occasionally used them. The times were lawless, and the country was wild and unsettled. These strangers were taken to be a couple of cowboys from the cattle range out for a deer hunt, so, when they entered Kelly's place, sat down at a table in the middle of the room, and ordered drinks, Kelly served them and thought very little about it.

Kelly's place was one of the best saloons in the country, having a big room, a bar running down one side, and a brass rail for your feet. Behind the bar a wonderful collection of bottles stood on the shelves, and a big mirror extended to the ceiling. Large kerosene lamps hung overhead, and the festoons of colored paper in loops from walls and ceiling (to attract the flies) gave a festive appearance. There were a dozen or so tables with chairs for poker playing, and a billiard table at one end. The floor was covered with sand, and spittoons were set at every table, as tobacco chewing and spitting were common practice. You entered the saloon through a broad doorway in which two small doors swung in and out, reaching only from a man's head to his knees, and opening on the boardwalk in front of the building.

As these men lounged about the table drinking, they grew more and more ugly. The raw whisky began to take hold and make them a little drunk. Then they began to boast of how they had "shot up a town," and told Kelly that the people of Silver Cup were a lot of skunks, and said they would like to see the —— —— sheriff of the place and tell him where to go if he horned in on their spree. Kelly kept his temper, for he was alone, and a row meant being killed by this wild and drunken couple. But he felt that trouble was sure to come soon, for these men were working themselves up to a point where they would get on their horses and go shooting wildly down the street.

Pretending to be beating flies out of the door so that they would not suspect his object, Kelly told a small boy who was peeking in at the wild men to run down the street and tell Mr. Smith, the sheriff, to come up, for these men inside were about to shoot up the town. The small boy found Smith, who asked what the men looked like, and the boy told him that they wore buckskin shirts and that he had heard them call each other Bill and Frenchy. Smith knew at once that these were the two men he had been warned against the day before by the letter from the sheriff of Black Mesa.

A Tenderfoot Sheriff

To his credit it must be stated that he did not hesitate a minute but, buckling on his two revolvers, at once walked to Kelly's Saloon. If he had not been such a tenderfoot he would have hunted up some men armed with Winchesters to go along and help him hold up these outlaws, but it seemed that he never even thought of it. A number of people noticed his slight and delicate figure as he limped past their cabins or stores and wondered at his intent look and pale face, but put it down to his feeling a bit ill. When Smith reached the saloon door, he stood a moment outside and listened. He plainly heard Arizona Bill say, "One more drink, Frenchy, and we'll show this —— of a —— of a town how to shoot 'em up."

This was enough for Smith, who felt that he must act at once, or in another moment they might come through the door shooting at everything in their way. He kicked open one of the swinging doors into the saloon to give him a clear view inside. There, at a table, sat the two men. Smith, before the door could swing back, aimed and fired both his guns. Arizona Bill jerked out his gun as he half arose from his chair, but he never fired. A bullet had passed through his throat. He stumbled and fell to the floor, choking. Frenchy got his in the stomach and fell forward on the table. But he managed to draw his gun and fire two shots at the figure of Smith, seen dimly in the cloud of smoke in the doorway. One bullet tore the sleeve of Smith's coat; the other splintered the door. Smith jumped back out of sight, and Frenchy, doubled over from his wound, made a rush for the door, stumbled across the walk to the street, and ran down it a few feet to a place where a gully made the walk higher; at this point he scrambled under the walk on his hands and knees to the far side near the building. Smith also jumped into the street and ran along looking under the walk. He did not know Frenchy was wounded. It was dim under the walk, but some sunlight came through the cracks between the boards, and soon he saw the crouching figure of Frenchy and saw his hand grab for his gun, which had fallen near him. Smith rapidly aimed and fired. For a moment there was silence. Then a thumping of Frenchy's boots as, in his last struggle, he had rolled on his back, and

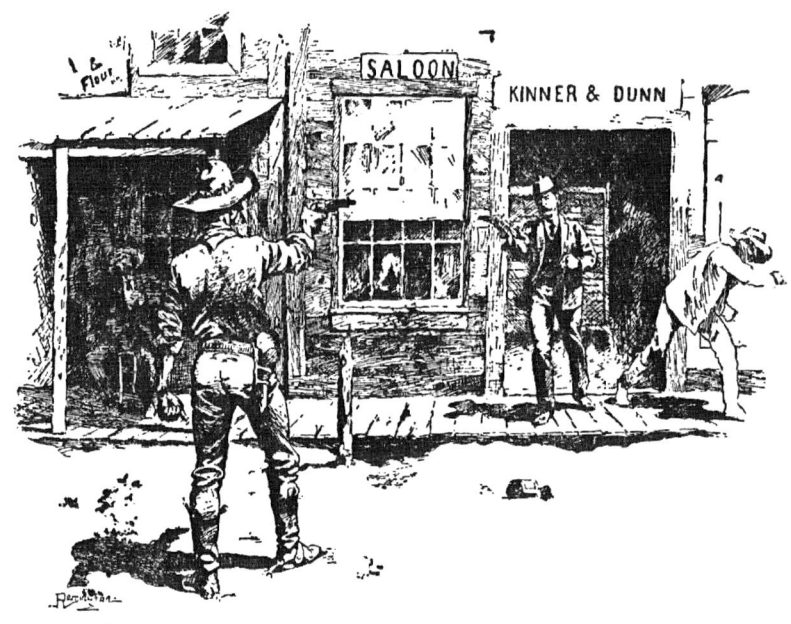

his twitching legs made his feet beat out a horrible "dance of death" on the under side of the walk. The knocks grew fainter, and ceased. Men crawled in under the walk, dragged the limp body out, and carried it into the saloon where they laid it out on the billiard table.

It was found that Frenchy had been hit first in the stomach and then, in spite of his wound, had run out and crawled under the walk, where the sheriff's bullet had hit him in one ear and gone through his head. Men came crowding into the saloon. In the midst of the confusion, Kelly, the barkeeper, came out from behind a barrel of whisky where he had been hiding to be safe during the shooting, and made a row over his billard table being all mussed up by a bloody outlaw's body. But, as most of the crowd ordered drinks and his business was booming, he was soon smiling behind the bar, serving drinks as usual. Arizona Bill lived only a few moments after being shot, and his body was put on the table beside that of Frenchy.

A Tenderfoot Sheriff

Some of the older men soon got together and made a kind of coroner's jury—far from legal—but it did well enough for the time and place. The clothes of the outlaws were examined. Nothing was found except on Arizona Bill, a newspaper clipping two years old offering a reward for his capture, dead or alive. It was agreed that the sheriff had acted within the law. A few objected and said that he had been "too damn quick about it," but, as he was a tenderfoot, this objection was passed over. So the incident was closed—but not until old Ike, the buffalo hunter, had his say. A tall stern figure he made. He was over seventy; his hair and beard were white as snow; his rawboned frame was still active and strong; the keen eyes were as steady as in the old days of Indian fighting and buffalo hunting. "I tell you all," he remarked, "that this is a showdown for Silver Cup. Them boys was bad medicine, but they ain't got none to grieve over them—no friends or nothing—and I say, let's give them a regular bang-up funeral and show that we all is for treating strangers generous." This sentiment met instant approval. The bodies were carried to a vacant cabin; old Ike was put as guard; and by unanimous vote, all poker games were to give their "kitties" that night towards the funeral expenses of the two deceased gunmen.

It was a night long to be remembered. The playing was high and furious, and in the cold dawn, the distant rumble of snowslides mingled with the songs and yells of the boys making a night of it.

The funeral of Arizona Bill and Frenchy will long be remembered as a red-letter day in the annals of Silver Cup. The morning was clear and fine, for a rain during the night had laid the dust. At an early hour a crowd collected on the street; in fact, many had not been to bed at all. There was none of the usual sorrow and gloom generally associated with affairs of this kind, but all seemed in a cheerful mood; jokes and laughter could be heard, and a spirit of holiday enjoyment was evident. The bodies, still clothed as when shot, were carried from the cabin and laid in the bottom of an empty ore wagon on some straw, as the nearest approach to a hearse. A couple of big mules were harnessed to this wagon, and as they walked slowly along three bells on collar and headband tinkled gaily.

Judge Jackson, on a white horse, appeared to be master of ceremonies. He had tied a big black handkerchief around his cowboy hat as a sign of mourning; and his red face, framed in his white hair and beard, shone forth like a full moon in August. The judge was a character and a favorite, but his legal knowledge was, to say the least, very faint and confused. It was also plain to see that the judge had made a night of it with the boys. He was barely able to sit on his horse as, at a trot, he ranged up by the wagon. Sandy McGee, a wild youth, the mirth of the camp, sprang into the wagon and settled himself down on the straw between the bodies, announcing in a loud voice, with a grin at the crowd, that he "was a-going to keep the stiffs from rolling about over the rough going."

For some queer reason it was decided that music must be provided, and heated arguments ensued as to how this important matter could be arranged. A piano was too big; an accordion was too small; at last the solution came, when it was remembered that Scotty, our shoemaker, had his bagpipes. Many had heard the doleful squeaks coming from his cabin, and Scotty was at last persuaded by a present of some fine old Scotch whisky to play for the funeral. In honor of his beloved Scotland, he now appeared in full Highland costume, his bonnet with ribbons, kilt and bare legs, and his pipes over his shoulder. Proudly he took his place in front, playing some tune he called a "Lament," that brought laughter and cheers from the crowd, and stampeded some broncos. At last all was ready, Judge Jackson gave the word, and Sandy from his gruesome place yelled, "Let her go!"

First came the usual collection of small boys—and all the cur dogs of course—then Scotty, blowing his best, followed by the judge and the wagon; some rode in buggies; some walked. A number of cowboys from the range country, out to see the fun, loped by the side. A few women in their calico dresses and poke bonnets trudged among their men down the street, over the little creek only a few inches deep at the ford, and then up

A Tenderfoot Sheriff

the hill to the mesa. At the end of the line a thin figure sat apart on a horse. His derby hat and dark clothes seemed out of place among this roughly dressed gathering. Sadly his eyes roamed over the motley procession in front. His face was sad and set, as if thought of his New England home with its stern and moral laws was out of place amidst the Western wilderness. His feelings were regret and sorrow that he had been driven by fate to kill these men, although no word was he ever heard to say regarding it. All knew he suffered in silence, and were not surprised when he soon returned to the East.

The cemetery near town was not to be used, for women with their children buried there objected to the outlaws' intruding on such sacred ground; so the mesa was chosen. No one was buried there. The way up the hill was rough. Halfway up, the wagon slued around and stuck; the mules balked; great confusion ensued. Everyone yelled, men pushed on the wheels, beat the mules, and cursed. Sandy from the wagon called for help to hold his stiff passengers from rolling together, there was much laughter and jokes at Sandy. Then the cowboys came to the rescue, riding their broncos in front of the stalled wagon, their ropes tied to the end of the pole and around their saddle horns as if dragging a steer. Their little horses crouched down, pulling for dear life. At last the big wagon heaved, rocked, and lumbered out of the mud to the top of the mesa on level ground, and, amid much excitement, at last drew up by the two graves dug by the Walch boys at daylight, in a shady place near a big pine. No more beautiful place could have been chosen for the resting place of these violent men.

The mesa, or "bench," as it was locally known, was a mountain park some two hundred feet above the town, extending for about one fourth of a mile in length and one hundred yards across—level, covered with grass and wild flowers, with big pines growing tall and stately in groves. It was more like the park of some handsome estate than the natural wilderness. The breeze made music in the tops of the pines; the sun filtering among the branches splashed the green grass with golden showers; paintbrush dotted the ground with brilliant red;

clusters of columbine nodded their heads in the shady nooks as the air stirred them. The sky was deep blue, without a cloud, and far off over a sea of dark green pine-covered mountains, the range of snow mountains cut the skyline and sparkled like diamonds in the sunshine. So peaceful it seemed that morning on the mesa, so near to nature and beauty, that it was a distinct shock to turn to the graves with the bare earth heaped up beside them, and to see those silent and sinister bodies, stiff in death, their bloodstained clothes crushing down the fragile beauty of the wild flowers.

The crowd now stood as if expecting someone to say a few words. A minister had been sent for at a camp fifteen miles away, but the messenger had returned to report that the minister had left for the East the day before. All eyes turned to Judge Jackson. His gray head shone like silver in the sun. He was assisted into the wagon where he stood swaying, held up by his friends. He was not a religious character, and the prospect of a talk evidently appalled and confused him. He hemmed and coughed, was heard to mutter, "—— if I can go it," and, half falling, was dragged from the wagon. A tense silence ensued. It was a tragic moment. Was Silver Cup to fall from grace in this last moment and be the laughingstock of all the mining camps for miles around, not able to pull off a real funeral after all the fuss and talk? All faces were anxious. Gloom and silence settled over the crowd, as with hats off they stood waiting. No one came forward. Failure stared them in the face. And then, as if by a miracle, the situation was saved. A little woman far back in the crowd, in a print dress, her poke bonnet hiding her face, commenced to sing in a voice as clear and sweet as that of a meadow lark, "Nearer, My God, to Thee." A thrill passed over the crowd. In a moment other women joined in the singing, and soon all were singing as if it were a natural thing to do. Old hardened sinners, their evil faces lighted up with long-forgotten memories of home, were soon standing with tears in their eyes.

No sermon could have been half as effective. All was as it should be, and the singing over, the men were about to carry the bodies to the graves, when the order of events was rudely interrupted, and turmoil broke loose again. A couple of our dogs, prowling around near the edge of one of the graves, suddenly engaged in a fight. In their struggles, they both fell into the open grave, from which arena there now ensued a series of growls and yells. This was too much for the sporting blood of the new West. Men quite forgot the funeral and, with eager curiosity, crowded around the grave shouting and pushing to see the dogfight, which was becoming a bloody affair in such a limited space. Shouts of "ten on the black," "five on the brown," mingled with the howls of the dogs; at last, as, pushed from behind, those near the grave dug their heels into the ground, one side of the grave gave away, and dogs and men mingled and struggled in the bottom. Men crawled or were hauled out; all bets were called off, and finally the bodies were in the graves, their big hats over their faces. Pine branches were thrown in, then dirt, and last of all big rocks to keep the coyotes from digging them up. After this was all attended to and the graves were smoothed over, old Tompkins, a carpenter, stuck a board up at the head of the graves, and on it he had painted in crude black letters, "Arizona Bill and Frenchy."

The crowd now scattered back to town. The ore wagon, filled with women and children, their voices growing fainter as they reached the edge of the mesa, went down the hill. All was still again. The graves of bare brown earth looked lonely in the shadow of the big pine. The trampled grass and wild flowers were slowly rising again to wave in the breeze, and, as the last of the crowd paused a moment on the brow of the hill and looked back at the graves, they saw a blue jay light on the top of the wooden grave marker, his long tail making saucy sweeps in the air as he strove to keep his balance. As if in scorn of man and his works, Nature had claimed her own again.

Chapter 7
A Fourth of July in Cowtown

I wanted a hospital where I could have my surgical cases in one place. A man permitted me to build on his lot on the main — indeed the only — street, a sawmill gave me the lumber, the boys helped me, and at last I had a shack about fifteen feet square, of unpainted pine. There were two bunks for the patients. The heating system consisted of a cookstove and a load of slabs for fuel. The plumbing was simple: a whisky barrel on the porch, filled with water, a pail and dipper.

Not much to make one proud, but in my ingenuous youth I did feel very proud of this hospital, and our entire population of some 150 adults greeted this addition to their town with much civic enthusiasm. The management of this institution was entirely in my hands, and, as surgeon in chief, superintendent, and general nurse, I felt quite elated. The financial strain was solved in a simple and practical manner by making a hard and fast rule that the patient who could stand on his feet cooked the food and nursed the other fellow who was bedfast. This arrangement had to be modified to meet unusual conditions, but as the average puncher received twenty-five dollars a month, was always "broke," and even in debt when he was admitted, the urgent need of strict economy in all departments was clear. In any case, the patients were cared for, often by volunteers from among their friends. So all was well, and everybody happy, which is more than can be said of some hospitals.

Probably I was a bit set up and "feeling my oats" over this hospital of mine, but my pride received a rude shock one morning. As I was going down the street to gaze at my small hospital, I was pained and grieved to find that some of my humorous cowboy friends had, during the night, amused themselves by painting all across the front of my beloved hospital, in large black letters a foot high, this touching tribute to my professional skill: "The shortest road to Hell," and amid a burst of laughter from some twenty delighted cowboys who were hiding to "see how the Doc took it," I was escorted to our main saloon and, needless to say, had to "set 'em up" for the crowd.

However, I passed over this bit of pleasantry and, before long, I had two patients installed. The hospital was filled to capacity. These first two patients were as different as human beings could well be; one was a Mormon from a new settlement of Latter-day Saints down in Utah, some three hundred miles south. He was about fifty years of age, all whiskers, and very dirty, ignorant, and fanatical, with a mean, sullen temper; my other patient, Joe Blake, one of the best riders in the country, was a wrangler for the L. O. T. on Rock Creek. He was a careless, happy-go-lucky youth with a mop of golden hair and a smiling face. One day while riding a "bad one" he was crushed against the side of the breaking corral, fracturing his right leg below the knee. I put him up in a plaster splint so he could hop about, and he quite cheerfully nursed the helpless Mormon, cooked the food, and did all the work. This ill-assorted pair were the source of much amusement. Joe took the Mormon as a huge joke, laughed at his cursing and ugly looks, and acted as if he were caring for a half-tamed bear. In the mornings Joe would begin the day by shouting out, "Wake up, Grandpa!" This would make the Mormon angry, and the flow of profanity and abuse would be answered by the merry laugh of Joe, as he lit the fire and cooked breakfast.

This Mormon had been shot in the abdomen and was in bad condition, but was improving. It happened in a curious way.

That summer, during the little rainy season, two of our cattlemen, one called "Hank," a long Texan, and the other a short fellow called "Shorty," were riding through the rain all over the range to find some horses which had strayed away from the night herd the night before. The rain came down all the morning, and it was cold, wet work going along the hogbacks and through the scrub oaks, looking in every gulch for the lost horses. A little after noon Shorty, who was in the lead, topped a rise at the end of a mesa and saw, below him, the valley with a river running through it, and could faintly make out, through the mist, the thin ribbon of a road that led to our town, some six miles up the river.

As Shorty peered through the rain he could just see a dark mass near the road, and while his eyes studied this strange thing below him, so hard to make out, he called Hank, who rode up and joined him. Hank, after one glance, said, "Looks like horses." So together they loped down the high bank to find out. As they drew near, a strange sight met their gaze. Four horses, still fast to the wagon, stood close together, all tangled up in their harness and unable to move. In their panic and struggle to free themselves they had cramped and turned the wagon half over. The load of oats, bursting the sacks, had tumbled out, and the oats were all trampled into the mud. As the boys circled around the wagon, they came upon a form huddled up in an old wet blanket and half lying in a puddle of mud and water. They knew by the shape that a man was under the blanket, but there was no movement to indicate that he was alive. They stopped their horses. Hank called out, "Say, stranger, what's the trouble?"

A low moan came from under the blanket. At once both men jumped off their horses, and Hank, reaching down, pulled a corner of the blanket away from one end, uncovering the man's head. They saw a wild, dark face covered with a mop of gray beard. The sunken eyes turned slowly up, looking at them as if dazed. The face was pinched and livid with cold. The whole body shook with violent chills. He could just mutter, "I'm shot."

The boys asked no questions but got to work at once. Shorty broke up a box from the wagon and had a fire going in no time, heated some water in a tin cup, put in a dash of whisky, and gave the wounded man a drink. After a little, the man told them he was a Mormon from a new settlement in Utah. He had raised some oats and was freighting it up the river to sell it. The weather grew wet, the road heavy, and his team played out, so he turned aside to camp and wait for dry roads. He was making camp and going to hobble his horses. He stood up on the hub of one front wheel and reached for his hobbles in the wagon bed. As he jerked the hobbles over the side of the wagon, they caught on his revolver, which was lying on them. The revolver was tossed up and, falling from the wagon, struck the hub at his feet and went off, and the bullet struck him in the abdomen. He fell to the ground from the shock of the bullet. The horses, scared by the shot, tried to run, and cramped the wagon around. He rolled off to save himself from the turning over of the wagon and the horses stamping about him. The blanket he had over his shoulders to turn the rain, stayed clinging to him as he rolled. He had been in this position several hours. The boys got the horses harnessed and the wagon righted and, with the wounded man groaning with pain, drove in to my place that night. I got the Mormon into bed at last. He was filthy—swarming with vermin—so I burned his clothes. I opened his wound in the abdomen (for in those old days we did not open a man up as we do today, but only enlarged the wound for drainage) and gave him opium. In a week he was much better, though still weak, and I felt that he was on the highroad to recovery.

As both my patients were doing so nicely and could take care of themselves, I started on July 1 for the big timber up north, on an elk hunt. At that time there were a large number of elk and deer in these mountains; there was plenty of grazing in the small valleys; many trout streams and lakes were scattered over this area; and the forests of pine and spruce, many of them large and stately trees, offered to the game a refuge hardly disturbed by man. This was an ideal place for hunting, for there were always grass, wood, and water. At that time it was a perfect wilderness, untouched by the ax of the lumberman and visited only by the Indian and the lone hunter. But in a few years the settlers crowded in, ranches were taken up, and game was driven out. I had a good hunt all alone except for my horse and dog. I had shot a big elk, but the horns were not very good. The night of July 5, I made camp in a little valley among some big pines and decided to leave for home in the morning. I had had my supper and was sitting by my fire smoking. Soon I became sleepy after the daylong hunt in the keen air. It was a dark night; all was very quiet; at times I could hear the stirring of the treetops far above me, my dog Czar lying beside me crunching an elk bone. The red glow of my fire lit up the stately columns of the big trees around me as if I were in some cathedral and, as I looked at the black night outside of my camp and thought how far I was from a human being, I felt a bit lonely.

Down near the little brook my horse was grazing, and I could hear at times the faint crunch of his teeth as he tore up a large bunch of the thick grass. The fire was dying down to a faint glow, so I unrolled my bedroll, and took off my boots—the only undressing I did, for at ten thousand feet with only two blankets, you did not undress.

As I pulled my blanket down to turn in, my dog Czar dropped his bone and, with a fixed gaze at one part of the dark forest, ran to my side. Every hair on his back stood erect. I suppose I was jumpy and nervous, being all alone in so wild a spot, far from people, and seeing no one for days. I had been warned that there was a band of cattle thieves somewhere in the big timber country where I now was. In any case I was thoroughly frightened. I caught up my rifle and made one jump behind the trunk of a big pine, to get out of the light of the fire. Czar lay by me, growling like distant thunder. At last I heard the snapping of dried branches as if some big animal forced its way through the undergrowth, and then a man leading a horse came into the glow of the fire. In an instant I had him covered. Aiming at his breast, I called out, "Stop where you are and don't move."

The man, to my surprise, went into convulsions of laughter, and called out, "Say, Doc, don't you know me?" and then I knew it was Smith, an old friend, so I had a laugh with him. As we sat by the fire he said, "Doc, that gut-shot Mormon down to your place has been took bad again, and the boys sent me up here to find you, and Doc, I certainly had a heck of a time following you." Smith was an old hunter, so he knew the hills and could follow a trail like a dog. In fact, it was Smith who told me as I left town where to find elk, and described the little park I was in as a good place, so he knew about where to look for me. He slept beside my fire, and we were up and away for home at dawn.

I found the Mormon in bad condition and could not figure out what had caused his relapse. Another suspicious thing was that Joe had twisted his splint all around his leg, and I had to put on another, but there was not a word from either of them as to what had caused these setbacks. They simply looked foolish and said nothing. Joe made a feeble attempt at a story of falling down the steps of the porch, but I knew by his guilty grin that he was lying, so I was patient, and waited. The Mormon grew better again. Apparently nothing could kill this sullen brute. I knew he had a .45 bullet in among his intestines, but he got much better, and by slow degrees I got the whole story that the boys were ashamed to tell me.

The Fourth of July in our place was a great event. This was the one day in the year when the town marshal just quit his job and went fishing, knowing quite well that he would have to kill some of his friends if he did his duty; the one day when a cowboy could turn loose for a high old time with no string on it. This Fourth, while I was away hunting, was a regular "humdinger," as all said. The boys came flocking in from fifty miles around. The saloon did a business unheard of before in the history of the town. Cattle were high at that time, and every rider had a wad of money to get rid of, so it was all the same to them; they were young, healthy as bears, and full of pep and ginger. As usual, on the Fourth, they ran foot races and horse races, rode "bad ones," gambled, got "full as goats," and rode around the town shooting holes in our iron stovepipes on top of the cabins.

As the day wore on, of course, a lot of the boys were well "lit up" and looking for some new devilment. The more timid citizens, seeing the likely outcome of this lurid celebration, wisely returned to their cabins, locked the doors, and crept under their beds until the frenzy died out. Late afternoon had come, and proceedings were calming down a bit, as a few of the most violent had at last been overcome by the rank whisky and were sleeping quite peacefully among the mules and horses in the town corral. Many felt a distinct relief that the worst was over. No one was hurt, and the boys had had their day of fun. Then suddenly, as if inspired by the devil, a half-crazy English ranchman came galloping down the street behind a pair of half-broken broncos, pulling up outside our saloon and standing up in his buckboard, swaying back and forth as in a drunken yell he called out, "Oh, I say, you boys, come and have some champagne—six cases, all on me!" Of course, the crowd accepted this free offering with unbounded delight. It appealed to their sense of humor that an Englishman should be sport enough to give them free drinks on the Fourth of July, and they crowded around the buckboard on foot and on horseback, while the Englishman, a little uncertain on his legs, stood up and opened bottle after bottle to fill the glasses, tin cups, and even pitchers held up to him. The general idea about this new drink was that it was a kind of cider—a mild drink fit for a Sunday school picnic, and great was the surprise of more than one case-hardened old-timer, when the champagne met the vile whisky that was in his stomach. As one remarked when he grabbed a friend to keep himself from falling, "That new drink sure has a kick like a steer."

Our one street now presented a scene like a circus parade. Darkness having fallen by this time, the scene was lit up by hastily made torches of kerosene-soaked rags on sticks that gave a lurid red light like a house on fire. The dust clouds from the trampled street rolled overhead like smoke, while the bang of revolvers and crackle of firecrackers, mingled with the wild yells that came from the drunken cowboys, gave the impression of a battle's being fought in the town instead of the fun-making holiday it was.

Our main street took on the aspect of a riot. A throng on foot and on horseback paraded up and down its length, making the night hideous with the noise. Small boys threw crackers under the restless and frightened broncos. Men danced around

A Fourth of July in Cowtown

in a circle, many carrying old oil cans that they beat upon with sticks. A few big cowbells were jingled. Revolvers were shot off in the air. As this half-drunken crowd surged up and down the street, my two patients at the hospital sat on the front porch enjoying the fun and looking quite restored to health. They had, I fear, had a few drinks, and the sullen Mormon, for once, was laughing and joking with the passing mob.

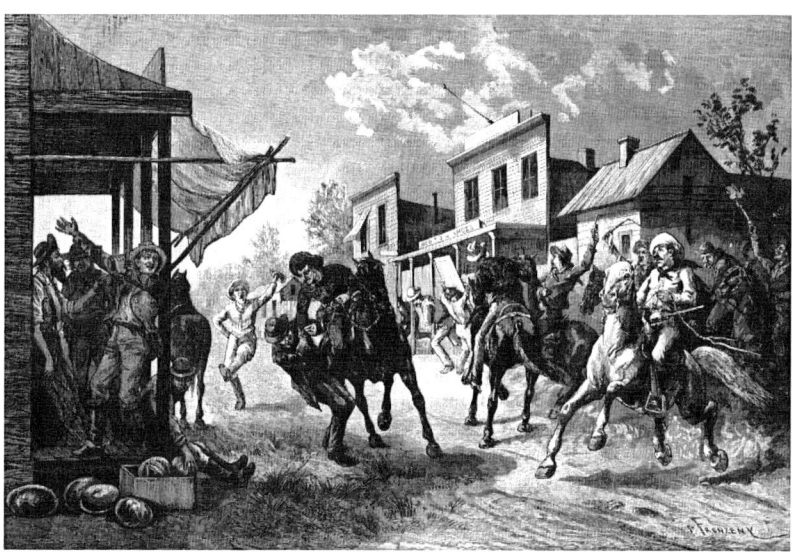

In an evil moment Shorty Davis, one of the wild ones, rode by my hospital, his horse jumping and crowhopping under the spurs, and Shorty, lit up by the champagne and natural devilment, seeing my patients on the porch, had a bright idea. Flinging himself from the saddle, he yelled to the world at large, "Say, boys, let's make the Doc's crips run a race." This perverted sense of humor caught the attention of the crowd in a second and spread among them like a prairie fire. It was a novelty, it was a good joke on the doc, who, fortunately, was not present. It had the taste, always so sweet, of forbidden fruit, and appealed to the drunken crew with irresistible temptation. So, in spite of the objections of a few more sober citizens, a dozen willing hands dragged my unfortunate patients into the street, the Mormon angry and cursing, and Joe, as usual, smiling and a good sport. A line was drawn by a spur in the dust of the street. Two lines of expectant and laughing spectators extended down the street, forming a lane to race in. The two men were made to toe the mark in the dust, Shorty standing ready just behind them, gun in hand. "Now, you lame ducks," yelled Shorty, "when I shoot, you run like rabbits."

Bang! went Shorty's gun.

Joe hopped along down the course with a stick. The Mormon ran a few feet, stopped dead in his tracks, and called out, "I ain't going to run."

Shorty, mad at seeing the race held up in this way, called out, "You run or be shot," and sent a bullet back of the Mormon's heels that threw gravel over his legs. The Mormon, with a fearful glance over his shoulder, saw Shorty aiming another shot and, with a shrill cry of fear and rage, darted down the street after Joe, and in wild leaps caught up to him.

The crowd went wild, surging along behind them, making and taking bets as they ran, and scrambling along, not to miss a detail. Suddenly the Mormon staggered, threw up his hands, gave a scream, and fell to the ground. He rolled over on his face, his legs twitching, and then lay like one dead. Many thought he was dead, but others bent over him and said he was breathing. Instantly the wild throng grew silent as the word passed along through the crowd that the Mormon was dead. A wave of reaction swept among them. The loudest mouths and toughest punchers that a moment before in a drunken frenzy were yelling the racers on, now stood sobered, with hanging heads. They had gone too far and, as realization came to their fuddled brains, a feeling of remorse and shame struck their reckless natures. They felt that it was not a square deal. The man was hurt, maybe dead, and they had not meant to be cruel in their fun. So when old Mother White pushed her burly form rudely through the crowd around the prostrate figure of the poor Mormon, her red face blazing with anger, her hands on her hips, the rough agent of wrathful justice, and proceeded to give a tongue-lashing to the ashamed boys standing around, not a man dared to meet her eyes or answer a word. In no time, under her stern orders, the Mormon was tenderly carried to my little hospital, where Mother White took charge and nursed him until I arrived. The Mormon did not pass out this time. What really happened to him with the bullet still in his abdomen, I do not know, but probably some adhesions were torn when he ran the race.

During the long recovery of this man, it was amusing and a bit touching to see the anxiety the boys felt regarding his recovery. I would be sitting in the hospital reading or attending to my patient, when I would hear the rattle of hoofs as a cowboy suddenly stopped outside, then his step on the porch, and his husky voice saying, "Oh, Doc." When I reached the door, a hand would crush a five- or ten-dollar bill into mine, and with a jump into the saddle, the visitor would lope away. Some were not so bashful, and after the usual donation would ask, "How is he coming?" and relieved on this point would remark, "You see, Doc, we was locoed by the new drink and we all never aimed to harm him none." And with this bashful confession of sin, off he would go.

A collection was taken up for the Mormon, his horses harnessed to his old wagon, grub for the trip put in, and when I said he could travel, off he started on the long drive to Utah—a huddled figure holding the reins, sullen and not answering a word to our farewell cheers. To my surprise, Hank rode after the wagon, not at all happy in his self-imposed task, but upon passing he drew up and stopped a moment to explain his motive. "You see, that crazy Mormon ain't safe alone, so I just guess I'll ride herd on him for a couple of days or so, anyhow until he passes the Big Muddy. He might be bogged down or something." And with a wave of his hand, Hank rode after the creaking wagon, to help a man he hated and despised. Good old Hank! So brutal and rough, so kind and true, so typical of his class that when in the spring Green River was in flood, and a cowboy was caught in the current, he rode in and pulled the man to safety. When the bank caved in, and Hank and his horse plunged into deep water where both were swept away by the cruel river, a gentleman in the rough was lost to the range.

Chapter 8
A Hoodoo Trip

In my early days I had to take some pretty hard trips, and suffer the usual hardships of long, lonely rides through the wilderness: poor food, snow and rain, heat and cold. I was young, tough, and, by daily practice, seasoned to it, and took it all as a part of my work, as the cowboys did.

But one trip I remember in detail because, as it happened, I had the luck to have as many things all occur in one trip as if some evil spirit were working against me. It was so bad that it actually became funny at times, and I developed a sort of grim humor as to what could happen to me next. I relate this as it actually occurred; it was bad enough without any embellishments.

Snake River was some fifty miles from our little cattle town, and some years before a small colony from Tennessee had located there. They were a "low-down lot," called "drifters," very poor, ignorant, and, report said, cattle and horse thieves. At any rate, they built a few cabins, had a few cattle and hogs, and lived as they always had. Cattlemen would have nothing to do with them and, in fact, often spoke of running them out of the country.

The road to the railroad ran by Snake River, and this summer a stage line was started from our place to the railroad. We were very proud of this stage line and felt that we were pretty near becoming a real town. There was a regular Concord coach with six horses and a change of horses every twelve to fifteen miles. When this stage came in loaded with mail and express matter, passengers crowded anyhow among the boxes and bags as it rolled and bounced along on its leather springs, the whole town of one hundred fifty inhabitants crowded in front of the general store and looked with delight and triumph at our link with the outside world. This pride was enhanced by the fact that the driver was our well-known townsman, Bob Hall, an old cattleman, and the best driver in Colorado. So when this summer evening the coach came to a stop and the dust cloud lifted a little, Bob stood up and, seeing me at the edge of the crowd, called out, "Doc, you're wanted at old man Hyde's place on Snake River."

I met Bob that night, and he told me he was making a short run the next day and would be back at Snake River in twenty-four hours on his return trip, and wanted me to go with him on the stage, for it would stop at the stock tender's place, only a short walk from Hyde's home. It was a change from riding horseback, so early the next morning we were off. I was the only passenger, and had the seat of honor next to Bob. I took only my surgical bag. Bob regaled me with the local gossip as we rolled along the rough road through groves of pines and cottonwoods, over little prairies thick with grass, and mile after mile with no sign of a ranch or a man. We saw deer on the hillsides as they broke away and bounded over the sage bushes as if floating, so easy and graceful was their motion. We watered at clear trout streams, fresh from the snows. The air was clear, the sun bright, and the blue sky without a cloud—nothing to warn me that this was to be a hoodoo trip for me.

Life was good, I was young, and there was no fly in the ointment until at the second change of horses. Here the stock tender was short of horses and had to put a mule in our swing team. That mule would not move. Bob beat him, the tender beat him, and their combined language was enough to singe his hair; but with legs braced, head and long ears shaking with his determination, that mule defied us to do our worst, until at last a rope was tied around his neck, the end fastened to the back of the coach, and we started. The mule threw himself on the road and was dragged along. I could not stand it. All his hide was coming off on the stones! So the tender cut him loose, and we went on with four horses. Bob was about wild, and I felt that the mule sent a hoodoo of ill luck as he lay in the road watching us with his sullen and revengeful eyes.

At last we reached Snake River. Here there was only a small, dirty shack where the stock tender lived, with a corral for the horses. As they were changing horses, Bob said, "Look out, Doc, them floaters is bad medicine. See you tomorrow," and was off in a rattle of wheels and a cloud of dust to make up lost time. The tender pointed out a low cabin down the river among some cottonwoods, and showed me the road to it. I asked him who was sick, and he replied, "I never took up with them Hydes none. I ain't heard nothing." Then I heard a few rifleshots and I asked, "Who is shooting over there near Hyde's place?"

"Oh, nothing, I guess, heard them shots all day; deer hunting, likely as not."

So I took up my bag and walked along the trail. Soon I was near enough to see Hyde's cabin—a tumbled-down-looking place, a pigsty up against one end, and a corral on the other. Smoke was coming out of the chimney, but the place looked deserted. All the wooden shutters were closed over the windows. The door, made of a dried cow's hide, was down; weeds and refuse were everywhere, while a couple of hounds were growling on the doorstep. Strange all was so quiet! I was at the gate in the fence around the yard, and was about to open it when, smack! a bullet struck a stone in the trail just behind me and whined as it flew off. The sharp crack of a rifle followed, and through the bushes I could see a puff of smoke float away among the pines on a ridge two hundred yards away, back of the cabin. I thought it was someone shooting at a deer. I gave a yell and waved my hat to show I was in range, and then another bullet crashed through the bushes beside me, hit the trail by my feet, and threw gravel over my boots. Someone was shooting at me! I was scared now, and pulling my gun, threw myself back of a rock by the gate. I was shaking, wondering who could want to shoot me. Then a board shutter was slammed back from a window of the cabin, a head came out, and a voice yelled, "You d—— fool! Bend down and run for it." I grabbed my bag, kicked open the gate, and, bending over under the bushes, I ran like mad for the doorway of the cabin. I hit the old hide door and fell against Hyde inside. It was so dark inside, coming from the sunlight, I could just see Hyde, a tall dim figure standing over me.

Now I was safe, and my fear changed to anger. I gave Hyde some straight talk about his letting me come and be shot at, without warning me. I wonder he did not shoot me. Here I was, about half his size, my gun still in my hand, shaking with excitement, and insulting this outlaw in his own cabin! He just stood there, a gaunt, sinister figure, holding his rifle, and waiting until I was through; then, very quietly he told me the facts.

I can see him now as he stood in the dim light, wearing a battered old hat, with his gray hair sticking up through the holes of the top. A white billy-goat beard hung down his chest. It was stained with tobacco juice, as were a few yellow fangs in his mouth, while his beard bobbed up and down as he talked. He said that he had had some trouble with the Becks, who lived back on the ridge, about a yearling calf. The Becks were "kin folks" of his, but there was an old feud between the families going back many years, and at dawn the Becks had opened fire and killed two of his cows in the corral. He turned the rest of the stock loose and returned the fire, but they were firing from the pines on top of the ridge, and were hard to see.

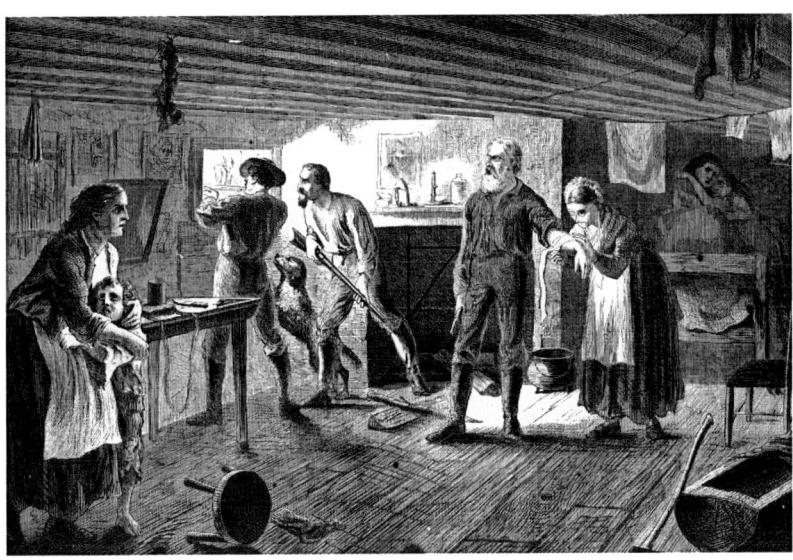

All day they had been firing into the cabin, but the logs were too thick to be pierced. He had no time to warn me. "Doc," he said at the finish, "them boys up there wasn't intending to kill you none, they was just calculating to scare you some. Why, them boys is mountain men, Doc; they could have shot the hat off your head and never touched you."

Well, here I was in the middle of a sort of family feud transplanted to Colorado. It all seemed so foolish and childish to me that I could hardly believe it, but I did not say so, as old Hyde was most serious about it. And it was real enough. They would aim to kill when the chance was offered.

Now I could see better, and looked around the cabin—a dirt floor, a low ceiling swarming with flies, a fireplace at one end made of mud and sticks, a bench and table, smoke from the fireplace, the shuttered windows making a dim light, and a lean-to with some bunks. I could see through a doorway, but the walls were thin and bullets had gone clear through it, so all had to stay in the cabin. By the fireplace a little old woman sat in a rocking chair, totally deaf. She kept rocking back and forth and noticed nothing. Evidently she was the poor old grandmother. By the fire, bending over cooking, a small, frail woman paid no attention to us. Her hair, tangled and uncared for, hung over her thin yellow face, her greasy Mother Hubbard was torn and stained, and her bare feet stood in the mud and filth of the dirty floor. She was a poor tired drudge of the wilderness, beyond hope or interest, but in a moment, looking over her shoulder, she spoke in a toneless voice, "Ain't he going to see Johnnie?" So this was the mother!

In my excitement I had forgotten all about the patient I was to see, and now, for the first time I heard muttering and low cries in a dark corner. There on a pile of skins and old sacks I saw a form covered with an old coat. At once I went over and lit a match to see better. There was a boy of fifteen. I asked for a lamp, and the woman lit and handed me one. I pulled the coat back, and held the lamp closer as I knelt down. One glance was enough! The swollen pustular face, the delirium, the fingers scratching at the face, and the smell, were enough.

Confluent smallpox! I had seen many cases like it before. I did what I could, put lard on the scarred and bleeding face, and tied the hands to protect the eyes. I told the family what it was. No one spoke. I was getting up from my knees when bang! a bullet hit the logs just over the boy, knocked out the chinking between the logs, and scattered splinters and dust all over us. In my surprise I nearly let the lamp fall; fortunately the bullet did not go through the logs. At this point the old grandmother piped up in a shrill voice, "The Lord will provide." What this meant I never discovered, but I nearly laughed out. The whole fool business was so mixed up with smallpox and a little war!

But Hyde flew into a rage. He grabbed his rifle and ran out of the door. Soon I heard the roar of his old Sharp's rifle as he let fly at his enemies on the ridge. I now ran out myself and, peering very carefully around the corner of the cabin, could just see old Hyde, flat on the ground behind a log near the corral, aiming and firing at the ridge. I was about to go back when old Hyde gave a yell, his old hat fell off, and he rolled over on his back. I forgot all about the danger, and was going over to him, when up he jumped and rushed past me into the cabin. I followed, and found the old man walking up and down, holding his chin in his hand, with the blood running through his fingers over his long gray beard, while he cursed the enemy at every step. I calmed him and washed the wound. The bullet had torn through the tip of his chin, taking a good handful of beard on its way. The wife now insisted on applying a cow-dung poultice to the raw wound, but I objected, and used carbolic and water. At last the excitement died down as night came, and to my surprise I was informed that the mimic warfare ceased at sundown, and a truce was called. Apparently there were set rules governing this ridiculous affair, strictly adhered to by both parties.

Hyde now watered and fed the pigs, and then there was supper, but the look of the food was enough for me, and with the flies in millions over everything, I could not eat. After supper old Hyde drew out an old, worn Bible and lit the lamp. The mother and grandmother sat by him, and he read several pages from the Old Testament—or rather he remembered them, for he could not read. Anyhow, the silence, the deep voice of the reader, and the simple earnest look on the women's faces touched me, although the aspect of the old villain, as, with bloody bandage around his jaw and his bushy hair standing straight up, he made fantastic shadows on the wall, looked, with his fierce face and weapons, exactly like a pirate of old. The family acted and lived the lives of their ancestors back in the mountains of Tennessee, and Colorado had not changed them in any way. Hyde was still guided by the "eye for an eye and tooth for a tooth" rule and, with his neighbors, was living up to it.

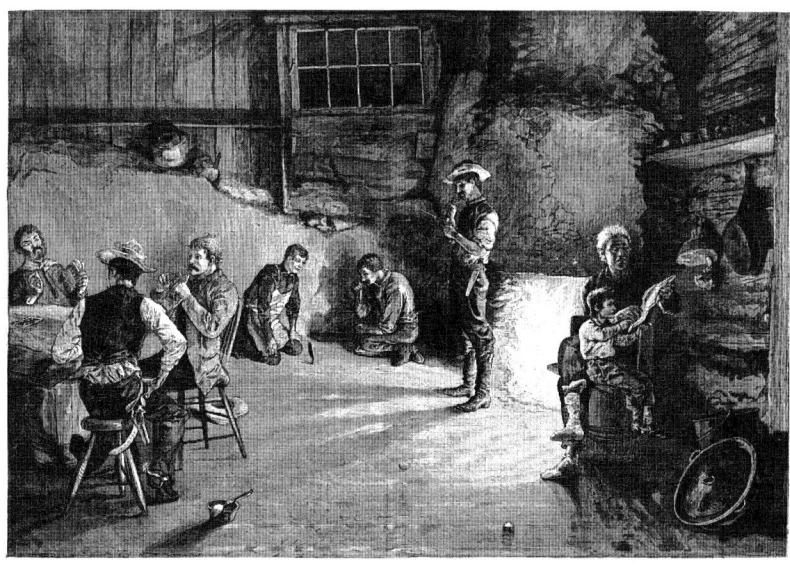

I felt as if I were living in another century as I saw these people at home. Hyde and the grandmother went into the bunkhouse, safe during the night. I lay in there until the bugs ate me up, and then I spent the night trying to sleep in the cabin on the floor, but the boy was crying out all night and rolling off his skins, so that I had to pull him back and help his mother. I gave him some medicine that put him to sleep finally, but the pigs grunted all night, and I was half crazy with bites, so gave up sleep and kept the fire going. I was glad to see the light of sunrise come creeping through the cracks in the logs.

I told Hyde I had done all I could and wanted to leave before the shooting began. I left some medicine for the boy, and by Hyde's advice I crept to a gully that ran down to the river. I kept pretty well covered, but had to dodge cactus plants that covered the bottom of the gulch; I got a few in my knees as it was. It was lucky I kept low, for before I was halfway to the riverbank, where I could be protected, I heard the snap of a bullet. Looking back, I saw a puff of dust as the bullet hit the dirt roof of the old cabin. So the clan had opened up hostilities again. I was glad to be out of it. I was soon under the riverbank and arrived safe at the stock tender's.

The stock tender at Snake River lived in a small shack, with a bunk and filthy blankets, the usual dirty plates, wood stove, and plenty of flies, but that bunk looked good to me, and I longed for it. My fear of infecting the tender held me back. The tender was called Dutch Charlie. Why, the grim humor of the West gave no answer. His real name was not Charlie, nor was he Dutch; but no matter—he had been so named by the crowd. I was much relieved when I told Dutch I had been with a case of smallpox, and that worthy replied, "Why, hell, Doc! I had it as a kid, so fire along." I slept until late afternoon, and woke up as hungry as a bear. Charlie, in the goodness of his heart, brought forth an aged box of sardines, his only delicacy, and treasured for some special occasion, so I ate all the sardines and also some sour-belly bread made by Charlie. I had just finished this banquet when up rattled the stage, all full inside, so I climbed to the top among the mail sacks and thrust my arms and legs under the ropes that held them, so I could stay on (for the stage buck-jumped over logs and ditches), and we were off.

Soon it was dark, and then we had a regular cloudburst. I had no slicker, and was wet through in a minute. Then as I clung amid the slushing cold water, I could hear the horses slip and fall down. The inside passengers climbed out in the mud, cursing and pushing the coach. It was stuck in the deep mud. At last Bob unloaded a lot of boxes from the boot in front, and the rack at the back of the coach, and left them by the roadside. Then we jerked and floundered along through creeks swollen by the downpour, up hills and down hills. Then the sardines, the generous gift of Charlie, got in their work, and I was so ill that nothing mattered for a time. At last I got rid of the sardines, and chill after chill shook me. Then the thought occurred to me that it was ten years since I had been vaccinated, and probably I would have smallpox from the exposure I had. Nice prospect, with the nearest doctor 150 miles away! At last the storm passed, and the full moon came out in a cloudless sky. We were up eight thousand feet and it was cold.

At last a light shone in among the pines ahead. This was sixteen miles from home—the last change, a log cabin and corral, the glow of a big fire showing through the doorway. Stiffly I climbed down, and soon was warming myself by a big log fire and drinking coffee.

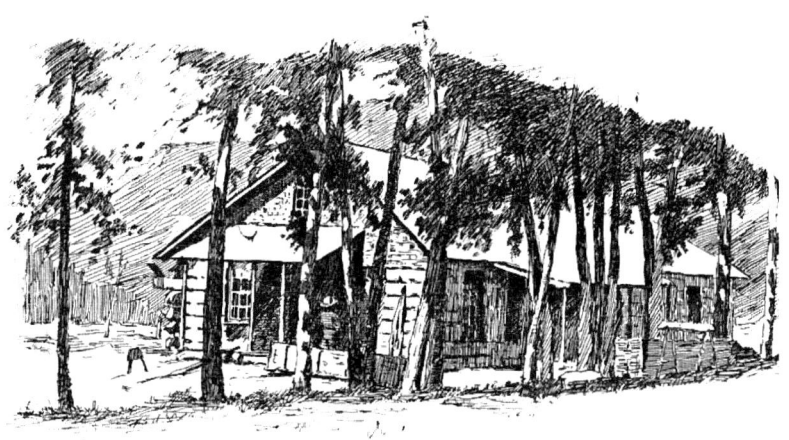

Then another blow fell. The sheriff seized all the stage horses for debt, including our six tired ones, and we were all afoot, with no room to sleep. I was determined to go home, and called the stock tender outside. Could he help me? Yes, he had a mule—a Spanish mule—in the little corral; and soon he quietly led the beast up back of the cabin. A pretty creature it was, slim and graceful, light grey, with big, kind eyes. With an awful saddle, held together by strings, but a nice gentle animal with a sort of amble that was as gentle as a rocking chair, I felt my troubles were over. Down the moonlit road I was carried easily and swiftly. It was a beautiful scene, light as day, so clean and fresh after the storm, with the tall pines throwing long shadows over the parklike glades. I lost myself in admiring its beauties, and in wondering if I could possibly buy this mule, so tough and yet so gentle, so easy to ride. And then without the slightest warning, and as quick as lightning, that mule gave a buck that was a terror. Straight up in the air she went, and then swapped ends. I remember going up in the air and seeing the moon rush across the sky like a meteor, and crash! I fell in a bunch of young pine trees. I lay a minute, my breath knocked out. Then the shrill braying of a mule rent the silence like a trumpet call, and there in the middle of the moonlit road was that mule, head up, braying in triumph. This was too much! I had been patient long enough, a plaything of fate. I groped around and found a heavy, solid, creek stone. I slowly crept up to that mule and, taking careful aim, I threw that rock with all my strength. I saw it strike just back of one long ear, and down went the mule, rolled on her back, and kicked in a feeble way.

I walked on, never looking back. The sun came up and dried my clothes. I strode on, and in time I reached "Hole-in-the-Wall," just as Jim Martin was hitching up to go to town five miles away. I slept until I got to my cabin. I went into the outside cellar where they brought me hot water, and I bathed in water and carbolic soap. I took off every stitch, hung the garments from the logs of the roof of the cellar, lit some sulphur candles, and let the bugs and smallpox germs fight it out. Then I went to bed and slept twenty hours.

I did not contract smallpox after all. Old man Hyde left the country for parts unknown soon after my visit, and never paid me. It was all part of the game in those days.

Chapter 9
A Tumor Clinic

I had heard rumors from time to time of a woman living at Sand Creek who had a big tumor on her head, under the hair.

Sand Creek, with only a ranch or so, was forty miles away over a very rough trail, and I never was called there. But some of my cowboy patients had seen her and urged her to come to see me. All I could learn about the case was that she was the wife of a ranchman, with grown children, and they all feared she was going crazy because she was so unhappy about the effect of the tumor upon her appearance. She would not see people, and kept indoors all that she could.

At last, one day in summer, I saw the Sand Creek family coming down the road to my place, just a little way out from the town. First, there was a wagon driven by her husband. The patient was inside under the wagon cover. Then came a regular cavalcade of mounted men and women. They had been three days getting the wagon over rocks and down timber, crossing creeks (in some places having to carry the patient), and they were a tired lot; so they were glad to pitch camp near my place on the riverbank.

A Tumor Clinic

Upon examination I found the woman had a big wen, quite a simple affair that any doctor could take off—just a gland in the scalp, swollen and filled with a cheesy matter. It swells the whole scalp, and is quite safe to operate. But this one was a giant among wens—as big as a coconut. It pulled the whole scalp to one side and came to the shoulder, so it certainly looked pretty bad. As I had not known what I was up against at first, I felt much relieved, and told them I would operate in the morning.

After supper I walked over to their camp and found my patient sitting up by the campfire, all alone, as the others had gone to town. She was still a pretty woman, small and delicate, with an intelligent face and blue eyes, and it was hard to realize that she had grown-up children. As she welcomed me and put a blanket for me to sit on by her, I was surprised to find that her voice was soft and refined, her English good, and that she was plainly of a better type than the usual rough pioneer. As we sat there we could see the sun going down in a red glow over the snows of the Continental Divide far away to the west. The river at our feet splashed over the stones, clear and cold from the snows, as it wound its way among the cottonwood groves on its banks. The trunks of the big cottonwoods looked like white marble against the pines on the farther bank. The silence was broken only by the ripple of the water and the rustling of the cottonwood leaves over our heads, as the night wind, cool and soft, gently stirred them so that they quivered as if afraid. A tinkle of a bell came from the night horse herd, grazing on the lush grass along the river meadow below us. A stick snapped on the fire, and the watchdogs growled under the wagon as the shrill yelp of a coyote came from the dark timber along a gulch.

Looking with sad eyes into the fire, she told her pathetic story. She had been very happy when, as a schoolteacher from Ohio, she had met and married her husband, a fine cattleman. But, by bad luck, he had lost out, and now, with only a few cows, they had settled at Sand Creek to try to better their fortunes. They were happy in each other and their children. Then came this lump on the head, growing larger and larger every year until it made her a sight to behold, and she shrank from strangers and at last even from her family. Though sure of their love and devotion, she grew ever more morbid in her lonely life, and at times even wished for death. All this was poured out to me quietly and without complaint, only the sad little face and the quivering lips showing her anguish of mind. As I looked at the figure by the fire, so worn and tired, so commonplace and yet so tragic, the plain, worn-out dress, the coarse apron, the thick clumsy shoes, the hands rough and red with toil clasped so closely in her lap, it all faded, and I saw only a very brave and gentle lady, facing a danger—unafraid.

I left her to the silence of the stars and the rippling river, and I walked away with a silent prayer that I might lift her burden.

Early in the morning I was in my office arranging for the operation. My office was in an open space not far from my house. It was built of adobe with dirt roof, to use as a fort during an Indian scare, when I wanted a refuge where I could not be burned out. After the scare was over I used it as an office. Soon, to my surprise, I found people coming over from town and making little groups around on the prairie, all very quiet and orderly. Evidently the news had got about, and in a small settlement all wanted to be on hand to help if needed.

My patient arrived with two women to help. Then the foreman of the L. O. T., a good fellow, made his way inside and, opening a window, said, "Doc, I'm a-going to tell the folks outside how things is going." There was no help for it! Young and nervous, I did not relish this relaying of my surgical progress, but I forgot it in a moment, and went to work. To my relief the first cut showed me there was nothing to fear. It was a cystic tumor, and quite free. My patient was a good sport; there was no cocaine, and no one to give an anesthetic, and she said, "I am all right, Doctor."

I had forgotten my friend at the window. He certainly meant well, but I should not have chosen him for a clinic reporter. His language was forceful if not technical, and I was a bit rattled when suddenly his voice rang out, "He's a-cutting into it." And a few moments later, "He's got it roped and hog-tied!" "She's a-doing fine, folks." "The Doc's giving her a drink!" This last was received by the anxious crowd with much interest, and a murmur arose, indicating their entire approval of my last therapeutic treatment.

As I bandaged my patient's head, my friend at the window concluded his efforts by announcing, "It's all over but the shouting, boys." This was welcomed by a cheer, and a few gentlemen who had endured the tension by the aid of a few drinks now discharged their revolvers in token of their sympathy and joy at the successful conclusion of the clinic. Of course, all crowded around, and my patient, a bit shaky, was assisted to her camp by many willing volunteers. Her husband was all gratitude, and, shaking my hand, said he "was broke," but "if I ever make it, you will have your pay, Doc." At this some of the boys cried out, "Don't worry, we boys can chip in and fix the Doc." When I told them I was only too glad to help the poor woman out, the excitement grew so intense that before I knew it we were all lined up in the O.K. Saloon and, as I did not care for alcohol in any form, I had to accept soda pop to show I was with them. At last I got away, when poker was started, but not before some of my friends were sound asleep and dead to the world.

My patient, with her husband and friends, left the next morning, and they did not go alone, for some of our boys went with them to make a better road and to help them over the bad places. My patient was another and a different being, all smiles and very happy. As she waved good-by to me from the wagon, I saw her face framed in the round end of the wagon cover, and so changed from last night—for now it was lit up with hope and bright thoughts—that I realized that my surgery had been but a small part, and that the real cure had been a mind cure.

A year went by. One day my patient's husband appeared and, to my surprise, was evidently on Easy Street. Driving a fine team and dressed in good clothes, he sprang out and greeted me most warmly. He said things had gone from bad to worse at Sand Creek until finally his eldest son had struck out to prospect over Gunnison way, and, as so often happens, youth and ignorance had succeeded by sheer luck where old miners had failed. At any rate, he had struck a rich vein, his father had joined him, and they had cleaned up and sold out at a figure that meant a fortune to them, and were now living in Denver. So I was paid my fee and, best of all, he said, "My little woman is as happy as the day is long."

Chapter 10
My Dog Czar

Late in September a cowboy rode down the street and about town, ringing a big dinner bell, and with a smile as if half ashamed of his job, called out, "Come a-running, all out for the winter herd." From stables and corrals all over town, horses and cows were driven into the bunch and herded down the valley to the lower country where there was little snow and good grazing. To keep a horse or cow during the winter cost money in feed, and they could do no work.

The valley was beautiful; a dozen high peaks, snow-covered to the green pine trees at timber line, surrounded us, and we could hear from time to time the dull rumble of the snowslides rushing down into the gulches—a wild and wonderful sight! Snow clouds rolled and tumbled upward as from a volcano.

The life was rough, men got drunk and killed one another, but in the main they were generous and kind. I was busy treating injuries and snowshoeing to the near-by mines to see cases. A dog would have been company for me, but I never chanced on one to my liking.

But one day a mine superintendent who was positive that I had saved the life of his wife (I was equally positive that it was an act of God) met me on the street and said, "Doc, I want to give you a real dog—not any d—— dog, but a crackerjack, half wolf, sent to my brother in Alaska from Siberia last year—a Russian husky, he called him. What do you say?" Of course I thanked him, and in due time the next summer, a big crate was hauled into town and backed up in front of Mother White's Hotel. Half the town had crowded around in no time, small boys asking, "Is it a bear?" I did not like the crate idea at all, for it looked to me as though the dog in the crate was no gentle pup, or he would have been led about; but I was told it was simply a precaution which was insisted upon by the express company.

The door of the crate was opened, and out walked my dog! He was a big husky, but with more wolf in him than is usual in a husky. He was covered with long hair, beautiful, soft, and curly, the color of sable, and under this he had a kind of thick wool coat. He had intelligent brown eyes and, as he stood erect and looked calmly around at the crowd, one at once noticed the quiet dignity and latent strength of the animal. He weighed about one hundred pounds and stood firm on his powerful legs. Every movement was slow and graceful. His great chest expanded as he sniffed the keen mountain air, and one could see by his attitude and every movement that his immense muscles were under perfect control and that, in a second, this quiet and dignified aspect could change into a tigerlike power, as quick and sure as lightning. One simply sensed the perfect machine in this animal, as with head held proudly up, he surveyed us with a gaze which showed no fear, but only a mild interest. I could hear the crowd around me gasp, as their eyes ran over the splendid build and kinglike attitude of this husky.

Soon a laugh went around the crowd as some town dogs pushed their way into our circle, all growls and warfare towards this stranger in their own town. The result was comical. Rushing in, all fired with combat to destroy this invader in their midst, they one and all stopped dead in their tracks as if at a signal of some psychic power, sliding along on their claws for a few feet, anxious only to stop at once, their faces a ludicrous mixture of fear and astonishment. I turned at once to see how my dog had so frightened them. He stood as if turned to stone. There was not a movement, not a growl, no baring of teeth, nothing but one curious action: the thick hair over his shoulders and back slowly rose and stood upright, increasing his size in a wonderful way, and giving an aspect so sinister and savage that we people who saw it, felt a thrill of fear creep over us. A strange and wolflike aspect seemed suddenly to emerge from the animal, transforming him in an instant from a calm dog into a beast of prey. It was all the more startling because it was so slow and deliberate; his eyes grew bigger and became fixed, seeming to shine like topaz jewels in the sunlight. As this hairy crest rose all along his back, like a warning a hooded cobra gives, it struck a certain note of fear in us. It was a menace so evident, that when the curs retreated and the crested banner of war slowly fell back to normal, we all felt a sense of relief. One old stage driver voiced our feeling, "Well, I'll be darned, if that dog ain't had me scart stiff!"

I took my dog home and, to be on the safe side, tied him up with a big collar and a chain to a staple in a log of my cabin, outside, where he could have fresh air. All went well at first. I fed him myself, but he did not make friends very quickly. I tried to be patient, knowing that such dogs are likely to be savage. But one day as I came back from a long ride, I dismounted and went to where he was tied up to see if he had water. I was dressed for the trail, in heavy clothes, chaps, and thick boots, with heavy gauntlet gloves. In my hand I carried my quirt loaded with lead in the handle. As I came near he sprang at me and bit me in the left arm. I jerked back, and the sleeve of my coat ripped off in his mouth. I staggered back and nearly fell. Perhaps I was wrong, but I felt I must master him then and there or I should be in danger as long as I had him. I was angry, and my arm felt broken where his teeth had closed on it. There he crouched, every tawny hair on his back straight up, his teeth bared, and his yellow eyes blazing rage and hate. The chain held him, or he would have torn my throat out in a second. I just closed in and beat him over the head with the lead end of my quirt. He grabbed my leg at the ankle, but the chaps and thick boots protected my legs somewhat. I am sorry now, after all these years, to think how brutal I was, and I wonder how we ever grew to love each other as we did afterward. I left him for dead and, while I limped into the cabin to dress my arm and leg, I was so angry that I hoped I had killed him.

In the morning I dressed in chaps and gloves and, with my quirt ready, made a visit to my dog. Huddled up against the log side of my cabin, he was a sorry sight. His head was swollen so he could hardly see, and as I spoke to him and laid down some meat and water for him, he made a move as if to spring at me again. I caught him a bad one with the quirt, and the fight was over. He was won, and I led him around and around the cabin. After some days I could see that he knew I was master, and when at last I took him with me up into the hills, where I shot and wounded a deer, he pulled the beast down. When I cut up the deer and gave him some of the liver, that settled it! I was the real thing in his eyes. As he looked at me, his muzzle all bloody from the feast, some primitive instinct was aroused in his half-wolf brain, and then and ever after I was in his thoughts the hunter, and he my devoted slave.

I had one fright. Czar was happy over a bone when my son, just able to walk a little, came suddenly around the cabin. Before I could move he had stumbled and fallen right on the bone between Czar's paws. I grew sick and faint. Horrible visions of my baby being torn to pieces before my eyes raced through my brain. I jerked my gun out, but dared not fire, for the child was too near the dog! And my baby, quite happy, was on his back, kicking his chubby legs up in the air, laughing as he pulled at the long hair on Czar's chest, while Czar, the savage wolf dog, was whining in a sort of caressing way, nosing and licking my child as if he were nursing one of his own puppies. I called to Czar, and he left the child, but as he came a few feet towards me, my youngster let out a yell for his new playmate, and back went Czar to the child, rolled on his back, and let the baby climb all over him, pull his ears and hair, in every way showing his love and devotion for my boy. So that was settled, but I was shaking all over from the shock.

From that minute he was my son's guardian. He followed him everywhere and, when I tried to keep Czar out of the cabin nights, he just stood at the door and howled for hours, so at last I had to give in and let him sleep in the cabin on a rug by the side of the crib. Often at night when all was quiet, a coyote would start howling down by the river, and I could hear Czar get up quietly and, bending over the crib, give my boy a little poke with his nose as if to say, "I am here, don't be afraid." As a guardian for my small son he was all anyone could desire. He adored the boy and, as I have said, let the boy pull his ears and tease him by the hour, never showing anything but a kind gentleness. But more than anything else did we appreciate his role of guardian angel when, too busy to have a baby underfoot in our small cabin, I devised a method by which the boy could be in the open air and yet be safe and not wander away. I buckled a big leather belt around the boy's waist, tied a rope some ten feet long to the belt, and the other end of the rope I fastened to a steel picket pin driven into the ground. Here, in the sunshine and on the dried grass of the warm prairie, with his toys on a blanket, my boy played by the hour, picketed out very much as we tied our broncos.

The boy was safe enough but for one thing, and that was the half-wild cattle from the hills that would wander down to the river at times. As my place was not fenced in, it often happened that two or three long-horned Texas steers, alarmed at something, would, without warning, come tearing by my cabin, and there was the boy right in their path. We had to keep watch every minute so as to rush out and herd them off. When Czar came into our lives this danger was attended to with energy and skill. He sat by my boy, and when any steers were headed our way, up he sprang and made for them, growling. With the hair on his back erect, and making his wild bounds at them, he was so like the feared timber wolf that the steers fled wildly away. Then Czar, all his fierce aspect changed in a moment, would come galloping back to baby to smell him all over to be sure he was safe.

At times, Indians on the trail to the north for hunting would leave their ponies and, squatting in a circle around my boy on the prairie, stare by the hour at the white baby; their gaudy blankets, feathers and silver ornaments, dark red faces, striped by blue and white paint, and small bright black eyes roving over the child, gave a weird look to my place. The boy was never afraid, but sat up straight and tried to say "How," as the Indians did, to their intense amusement. But with Czar it was a different story. Restlessly he prowled around the boy, and when some young brave came a little closer to see the boy better, there was a rush of a big tawny dog, who, with bared fangs, growling like a thunderstorm, advanced with such evident anger that the boldest brave quickly drew back. So we felt quite safe about our little boy, tied to a picket pin, playing long hours on the dry prairie in the Colorado sunshine.

When the snow and cold came in the fall, Czar's delight was unbounded. Dashing into snowbanks, he rolled in the snow and seemed to say as he barked at me, "I tell you, Master, this is the country!" He was a true snow child, and never tired of it. When the snow grew too deep, I had to make my professional trips on skis, as no horse or man could break a trail through six feet of snow. I was worried whether or not Czar could come with me, and I knew it would break his heart to be left behind. He could not flounder through the snow and keep up with me on snowshoes, so I thought, but he did! He just trailed in behind me. As I slid along on my snowshoes, I left two narrow trails near together where my snowshoes, or skis, had pressed the snow down. Along these narrow trails Czar soon learned to walk. I would tease him sometimes by straddling my shoes far apart; and poor Czar could not keep his balance on one ski trail. Plump! he would tumble into a soft bed of snow, buried up to his ears, and barking for me to help him out.

Later in the winter a crust formed on this deep snow, and then Czar could gallop all over, the crust bearing his weight. One day an idea came to me — why not make Czar tow me along on my skis? I stepped along on my waxed skis almost as easily as in skating, so I tied a line about fifteen feet long to his collar. He took to it at once, true sledge dog that he was. Then we had a grand time. Along came Czar at a gallop, and, holding the end of the rope in my hands, all I had to do was to keep my balance and come sliding over the miles of snow without effort, at a speed I could never hope to equal alone. Much surprised were people at some of the mining camps when, looking along the trail for the doctor to come, they would see my big dog come racing along at top speed, his tail curled well over his back, barking to show how proud he was, and then, a few feet behind him, erect and only holding the rope, the doctor flying over the snow as if by magic.

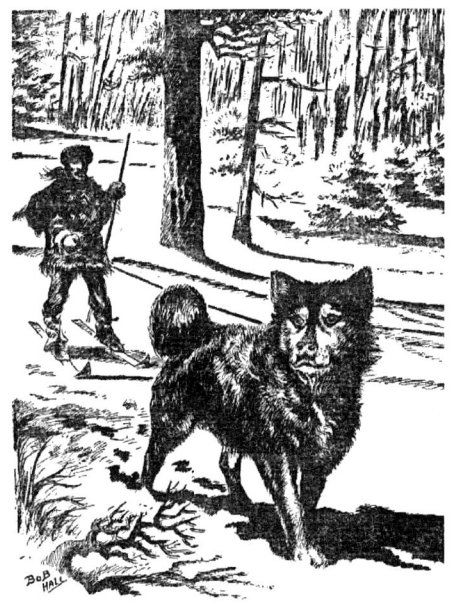

It was not always so easy as this. Often the trail led up a big mountain, and then the pulling was too hard for Czar, and I had to plod ahead with brakes on my shoes to avoid slipping backward. I used a piece of deerskin under the middle of the skis as a brake, the hair pointing backward. Often at the top of the mountain there would be a long slope free from rocks or trees for a few miles, the white plain descending several thousand feet, and here I would start off on a long slide. As I gained speed, the wind whipped by me with a shrill whistle, and long snow plumes flew off from the front of my skis and floated away behind me like white smoke. I must have gone forty to fifty miles an hour on these long slides. Back of me would come Czar, racing like a good one to catch up, and barking for me to slow down.

In another way, also, Czar was of real help to me. Some miles from town there was a gold camp located on a bench about fifteen hundred feet above the valley. There was a trail leading to it that could be used by burros, but only for three months in summer. In winter the snow was too deep, so a trail was used that went up the face of the mountain by long zigzagging back and forth across the almost perpendicular wall—a trail, narrow and dangerous at the best of times, very slippery, where a fall meant a plunge down hundreds of feet to sure death on rocks below. This trail was a real terror to me. Even in daylight and fine weather it was one to make any climber anxious, but with zero weather, a high wind to drive the drifting snow into the eyes, and on a dark night, laden with a pack of my medicines and surgical instruments, there were times when I wondered if it were worth it. But I knew that at some small cabin above me there was a man in real need or I should not have been sent for, and so on I would go, crawling like a fly, the cold and altitude knocking all the breath out of me as, step by step, I worked my way up and up for maybe two or three hours. There were no trees or bushes—only bare rocks and snow, and very often snow slides went crashing down to the valley below.

One night they called down from the mine at the top to a family living at the bottom, that a man had crushed his leg and a doctor must come, so they called me, and I snowshoed over, left my skis, and started up. Czar was with me. I was half sick and felt weak and unfit for the trip. About halfway up I felt pretty ill, but all the way Czar would run up that steep trail as if it were level ground, his splendid muscles and brass lungs making nothing of it; and way on ahead I could see him sitting on the trail giving short, impatient barks as if to say, "Hurry up, Master, this is fun." Wearily I plodded after him, panting and about all in. When I reached him one time and flung myself down beside him for a moment to get my breath, a sudden thought occurred to me—a brilliant idea, but would it work? I said, "Czar, you will have to help me up this infernal trail." I then with both hands just caught hold of his bushy tail, near the end, and called out, "Go on, Czar!" That dog had sense! He caught on at once, and with strong, steady steps, he pulled me up that trail as if he had been a horse. I could pull back as hard as I wanted to, it made no difference to him; his strength was wonderful. He never slipped, but just towed me up the terribly steep places as if I had been a child. It was nothing at all to climb this awful trail with Czar pulling me, and, best of all, he was so proud of doing it that when we reached the top he capered all about the miners there and barked and barked to tell them how he had done it!

It was, however, as my companion on my hunting trips, that Czar showed his intelligence, courage, and strength. Not at first, because the latent wolf in him caused him to rush at a deer and chase him until, hours later, he returned, leg weary, his coat torn by the bushes. Gradually, by holding him in leash, I taught him as soon as game was sighted either to creep silently behind me or to lie at my feet, and then, if I shot and only wounded a deer, he would, at a sign, bound forward and bring the deer to bay or throw him until I came running up to finish him with another shot. There was plenty of game in the mountains in those days. Both deer and elk came down in the fall after the first snow, to the better feed in the lower valley. We would kill a few, pack them in, and hang them up on the north side of our cabins. When frozen, they would keep all winter. It was for food that we hunted, not merely to kill, like the tenderfoot.

One fine day in the fall Czar and I went hunting. I left the horses roped out in a good place, and we hunted on a mesa, a wild and beautiful place with long stretches of tall grass, thick groves of white aspens very like canoe birch, and a few stately pines, with a clear stream, full of trout, wandering along through a region so like a gentleman's park that it was hard to believe it an untouched wilderness. Carefully we crept along, taking our course over game trails that wound along through the meadows and trees. Suddenly, in a little glade, I saw three deer—a big buck and two does. The wind was right. I sank behind a group of trees; Czar crouched at my feet, shaking all over with excitement. I noticed the distance—about seventy yards. The buck would feed with his head down; then up would come his head as he looked all around for danger; at last he looked about and turned a little so I could see his shoulder. I took careful aim, but just as I fired he twitched his shoulder at a fly bite. The smoke hid him for a moment; then I could see he was down with his legs kicking in the tall grass;

My Dog Czar

then all was quiet, except the crashing of bushes as the does ran through them.

Czar was whining, anxious to go to the buck, but I made him stay by my rifle, and with only my skinning knife in my belt, I walked over to where the buck was lying. He seemed dead enough to me as I got nearer to him. He was on his side, still as death, the long grass around him standing straight up with no motion. As I got closer I stopped a moment to see if his sides heaved in breathing, as I knew the danger a wounded buck could be; and then so suddenly that I was dazed, he gave one kick, and with a bound was on his feet, snorting and stamping the ground in a rage. In another second he saw me and charged. I just turned and ran as hard as I could, yelling for Czar at every jump. I could hear the buck slashing through the tall grass, just at my heels; and then he struck at me with his front hoofs, just missing me. I gained for a moment, but he was just behind me again. I could feel his hot breath stir my hair, he reared and struck, caught my shirt as it curved out behind me, and tore it loose at the neck, staggering me so that I nearly fell in the clinging grass. I was about done for, and felt my legs giving away. Another stroke of those sharp hoofs and my head would be cut wide open to the bone and my body would be stamped on and stabbed by those sharp horns. All my breath gone, stumbling and about to fall, I felt a rush through the air close to me, and the brown body of Czar tore by. I heard a heavy fall and looked back. Czar had missed the throat of the buck and was rolling over and over. The buck came at me again, as mad as ever, and instinctively I drew my knife, but Czar was on his feet again, and, bounding up just as the buck was about to strike me, caught his throat in a wolf grip. Both fell, the buck pounding Czar's head until he was covered with blood. I ran over to my rifle, caught it up, and ran back and shot the buck through the heart. For a few moments I fell down and felt faint. Czar was growling and savagely jerking the dead buck all over the place. I first called him off and then examined the buck. My bullet, a .44 Winchester, had hit the base of one antler close to the head, as a streak of lead showed, and then glanced off. The shock had stunned the buck for a few moments, and, as I drew near him, he had suddenly recovered.

I sewed up Czar's head wounds, and when I cut up that buck, Czar had the best parts of the liver.

At another time Czar was my good angel. I was called to see a man on a ranch forty miles away, over a country unsettled and wild, with only a faint trail leading across it. It was October, and at six thousand to seven thousand feet the weather in the fall suddenly changes to winter. I knew this, but was careless and did not take my skin coat. I took an extra blanket, and with a saddle blanket felt that I had enough clothes. I also took some bread, some chocolate, and a tin cup; this with instruments, medicines, and rifle made, I thought, an adequate outfit. We started early, Czar bounding along, glad to go, jumping up to snap at my pony, and racing every rabbit.

It was a warm bright day, almost like summer. At noon I watered my horse at a creek, had some bread and chocolate, and felt sure of reaching the ranch before dark, but when we were about halfway, riding on through rather a bare country, I saw a dark cloud coming toward us. The air grew colder and colder, while a fierce wind sprang up; it grew quite dark, and snow in the form of sharp crystals lashed in our faces. I knew what it was—a mountain blizzard! The wind seemed to cut through my clothes like a knife. The snow blinded me; I lost the trail; my bronco would not face the storm. Every minute the wind grew stronger, and the cold more severe. There was no shelter, for the nearest timber was miles away. I got off and led my bronco up a side gulch. There was very

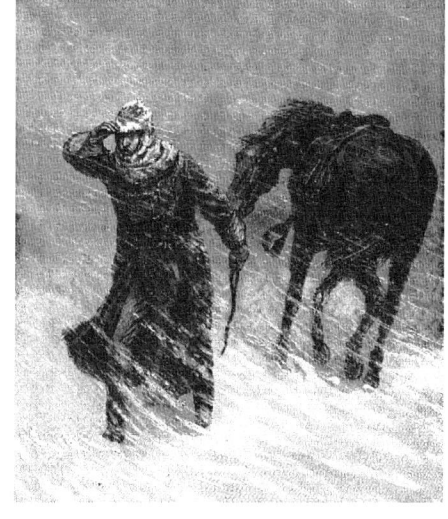

little shelter. The gulch was small, with nothing to make a fire but sage bushes. If only I could reach the timber! But we could not move a yard farther. I took the saddle off my bronco and turned him loose; he would freeze on a rope, but could shift for himself. Then I made a fire, after much effort, for I had only sage bushes, and the wind would blow the hot embers away all the time. At last I heated some stones in the fire and sat over them with the blanket over my head. I had to walk around and pull up bushes to keep the fire going. In timber it would have been easy, but these sage bushes were burned up in no time.

As night came on, I was losing strength from the constant hunting for bushes and the exposure. My teeth chattered and, though trembling and growing sleepy, I realized my danger. There were no dwellings for twenty miles. I could not make the thick pine timber a mile away, for no one could live in that wind. It was as dark as pitch, and blowing so hard that the snow was not deep enough that I could crawl into a drift as I had done several times before when caught out like this. I found it quite comfortable and huddled over the hot stones in my blanket. The fire was out. I wrote a note to my wife in my history book. I could not see, just wrote by feeling. I called Czar, and he came over and sat by me. This child of the cold and snow was protected by his long coat and undercoat of wool. He often slept all night out in the snow. I put my arms around him, and how warm his big body felt! I had an idea. I pulled him into my arms and drew the blanket all over us. It was a big Indian blanket, a Navajo, and thick; it turned the wind off like a board. Czar struggled at first, until I let his head out into the air. Then he seemed to understand, and soon was sound asleep.

The comfort of that warm body seemed to go all through me to the tips of my toes! I was more hopeful now, but the night was very long before me. The wind was fierce, and it was with difficulty that I held the blanket around us. The wind howled and tore at us, and I was cramped and tired; but sleep was dangerous. Once Czar had a nightmare—fighting a wolf, I suppose—and kicked everything over. I nearly lost the blanket, but caught it just in time, and when we settled down again I was shaking so that Czar kept licking my face trying to see what the matter was. I talked to him, and soon he was asleep.

It seemed a year, but at last it grew light. I could not stand, I was so cramped and cold. Finally I gathered some dry bushes and made a fire. The storm grew less, and at last the sun came out. I was warmed a little, but still felt weak and shaken. I noticed my left foot seemed dead, and pulling off my boot and sock, found it white and frozen, like marble, with no feeling at all. I feared I might lose it, so started at once, stumbling and limping down the rough gulch to the trail. I must have my bronco. I called Czar, and Chum, my horse, waving my arms around to tell Czar to search. He understood and was off at a lope, circling the hills. In less than an hour I could hear him barking, and then over a hill came Chum toward me. My horse was safe, for a native bronco can weather any blizzard in some gulch. I soon saddled up and made good time, reaching the ranch about noon. The cowboys there were as kind as possible. I attended to the patient, and then to my foot. I had a bad time with that and nearly lost it. The toes all grew black. Being a doctor and knowing what to do was all that carried me through. It was five days before I could ride home, and then two of the boys insisted upon going with me. Czar, the hero of the occasion, was much made of, and I feared he would be killed by kindness, as all the men fed him.

That it was a close call for me, and that the blizzard was a bad one, I had ample proof on my ride up the river. We saw many dead cattle; in one bunch of bodies we counted fifteen. They had drifted with the storm against a wire fence and had frozen. Two cattlemen I knew, Tom Blake from the Lazy T outfit and Charles Sommers, a horse wrangler from Green River, were found frozen to death not five miles from where I had been caught, and I was more than grateful on this return trip, as safe and warm in the sunshine, I rode along and watched Czar, who bounded on ahead of me, turning now and then to see me, and barking at me as if to say, "I saved you, Master." Then I remembered the long dark hours, the bitter wind howling and tearing at the blanket, the cold growing worse every hour, until it seemed to pierce my vitals and dull my brain. I thought of the horror of such a death with no help near, and then of the big shaggy dog in my arms, his warm, vital body giving me comfort and renewed strength to carry on, and how, at times, he would raise his head and, half asleep, lick my hands and face as if to say, "All right, Master?" No wonder I loved him. And yet I lost him — a sorrow I can still feel.

We were on a little trip to a ranch ten miles away to see a sick child, on a sunny winter's day. My horse, Chum, raced Czar over the prairie, happy and alive in the keen air. I saw a dead colt at one side, his skin slashed, and I knew he was poisoned by strychnia as a trap to kill coyotes. I called to Czar, "Keep here, Czar!" He seemed to come with me, but I forgot him in crossing a rough gulch. Then I missed him and whistled for him, as I stopped and faced around to watch the back trail. Then in a moment I saw him coming along with his powerful lope, jumping the sage bushes in his path with his smooth and graceful bounds. He nearly reached me, jumped a sage bush, seemed to stumble, then to recover; and then he had a convulsion. His jaws locked, his head arched back, and his legs grew stiff. I jumped off and went to him. He recovered a bit. His teeth chattered, and his muscles all quivered while his breath came in harsh gasps, his sides heaving to get his breath. He crawled to me, pushed his head against my chest as I sat on the ground, gave one look, soft and gentle, out of his brown eyes; then a terrible convulsion seized him and he was dead. I sat stunned. At last I gathered rocks and piled them on him to keep coyotes off. I cried as I rode away. There was nothing I could have done. There was no lard or chloroform — nothing. He had had a drink at a creek a few minutes before and, no doubt, had a big dose of poison which became active with water in the stomach.

I went back the next day and carried the body on a sled to my cabin, where I buried him in a sunny corner where he loved to lie.

Chapter 11
Rough Surgery

I built my log cabin on the bank of our river, in among the cottonwoods, and a quarter of a mile from the little cow town, partly to have quiet—not to hear, night after night until small hours, the music of the fiddle and piano, and the voice of the man who called out, "Make your bets, gentlemen!"—and partly because our river meant much to me, coming as it did fresh from the snows on the high peaks of the main range. It ran over a bed of sand and round stones, clear as glass and, in the quiet shady pools, under the bank in the shade of the cottonwoods, one could see the big trout whisk their tails as they looked for grasshoppers or flies to fall on the smooth surface above them. With a gentle splash and musical murmur, the stream flowed past my cabin so quietly and peacefully that I grew to love this voice of the water, and in my bed at night it seemed to say, "Rest. All is well."

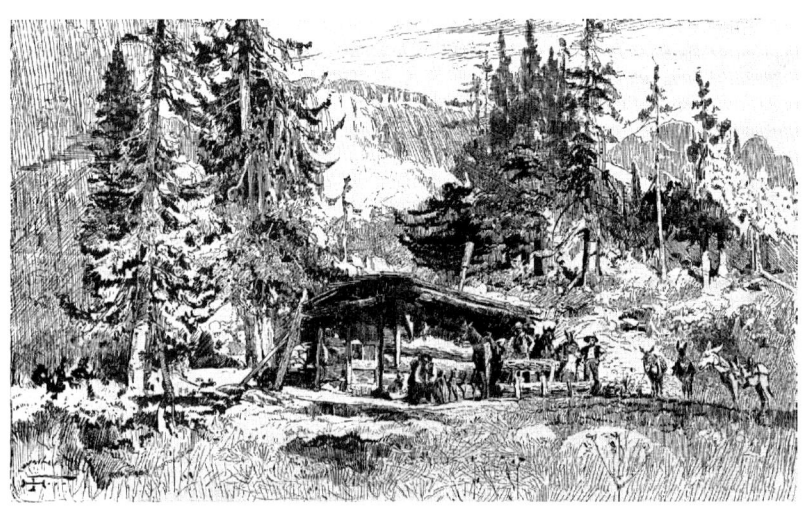

Rough Surgery

This morning as I sat quietly on my porch watching the river, on the other bank came a doe and a fawn. Timidly, with short steps and many a halt to listen for danger, they reached the water. Wading in a little way, they drank deeply but still fearfully as, with dripping mouths, they would suddenly stop and lift their graceful heads and pointed ears, while their beautiful eyes would swiftly scan the banks for any sign of an enemy. I kept still and enjoyed the picture, as the little spotted fawn, at such times of alarm, would crowd close to its mother as if seeking protection, and then the doe would bend her head down to her baby as if saying, "I am here. Fear not."

Suddenly the gallop of a horse on the planks of a bridge over a little creek behind my cabin broke the silence. The doe and fawn gave one jump and were gone like a flash of light. As I stood up and walked around the cabin there was a man on a bronco loping toward me. They suddenly drew up not ten feet away, scattering the gravel as they slid along, and the man, without a word, unchecked and threw the heavy stock saddle on the ground, as any good wrangler would, to give his bronco more air. And this bronco needed it, for he stood, covered with lather, his legs far apart and his breath coming in gasps, his sides heaving. Then, as the man led the bronco to the shade under a tree and came closer, I knew him as an A-Bar-A man called "Sandy," but what with alkali dust hovering him and with his handkerchief tied over his mouth, I knew him only when he spoke to me.

"Doc," said Sandy, "Frank Scott was shot at sunup by that rustler, Bob Kelly, in the Bad Lands about ten miles east of the second ford. I left some of the boys with him. I came a-running, got a fresh horse at Blair's, and am going to get me some grub and a bedroll, pack a horse, and then will come right after you. We ain't got nothing down where Frank is at."

I knew the place—a stretch of bad land down the river. There was no water, no wood, no grass, only greasewood, cacti, sand, and hot rocks. Sandy helped me saddle and pack my things on "Funny," my little pack horse, and away I started on the cowboy trot that eats up distance and does not tire the horse.

I had found, by rather hard experience, that to go on a trip such as this, along trails and through a wild country, without a cabin or camp being seen for many miles, one should be prepared to make a camp if necessary, have a bed and some food, and the means to live alone for several days at a time.

After some study and many experiments, I bought a pony from the Indians, taught him to carry a pack and to follow my horse like a dog, day or night. He was rather small, but sturdy and tough. The Indians had slit one ear as a kind of brand, making him look funny, so I called him "Funny." I made a packsaddle myself, just to fit him, and panniers of elk hide to fit on each side, one to hold my surgical kit and medicine, and the other for my provisions and cooking things. On top of the packsaddle I put my blankets, a small pillow, and a thin mattress, all rolled up and covered with a canvas sheet to keep out the rain and to cover my bed in bad weather. All was made fast to the pony by special cinches, breast collar, and breeching. So I had with me on this pack everything I wanted, and could be comfortable, warm, and fed, even in winter.

I followed the trail along the bank of the river, at first through a beautiful country of long stretches of meadowland, with groves of cottonwoods, their vivid green leaves trembling in every breeze—as if the old legend of the Spanish were a fact—that the true cross was made of cottonwood and the leaves were still trembling with sympathy and sorrow.

The wild flowers showed bright splashes of color amid the green grass of these little prairies. Columbines, paintbrush, and little sand lilies were growing with no eye to see them. I saw herds of deer bounding and flitting away as I rode through the groves of trees. The whole scene was as it had been for centuries.

Some fifteen miles down I stopped at Blair's. Blair was a dirty brute, married to a squaw as dirty as himself, living in a tumbled-down little shack, having only a few horses, and making his living by trading with the Indians. Here I took off both saddles and rubbed the backs of my horses, tightened up cinches, and prepared for the travel below, as Blair's was the last place for many miles where men lived.

The country now became more barren. Trees disappeared; only a little grass was left at the river's edge. All the rest, as far as the eye could reach, was a wilderness baking in the rays of the burning sun—a country of stone buttes, dry gulches, hot rocks, sand, a few clumps of sick-looking greasewood bushes, and cacti everywhere, waiting with their sharp spines to pierce the man or animal who touched them. As I looked over this desolate and savage region extending for miles on every side, the wind would lift up the sand and whirl it away in fantastic shapes, glittering in the sun and twisting like some gigantic serpent in pain. In places the patches of alkali covered the ground with a white glare like fields of snow; a terrible place to be wounded in, and I thought of Frank Scott, away off in that arid waste, waiting for me, and I hurried my horses on.

As I looked at the river beside me I could see that it was now becoming cloudy and was gaining in depth and swiftness, while giving a roar over the rapids. The snows were melting on the high mountains, and the river was going into a flood. I was now near the upper ford and must hurry if I were to cross to the east side, where Frank was. I could not risk keeping on to the lower ford as Sandy had told me to, for it would be too deep to cross with this flood coming down; so I hurried down to this ford. The river was one hundred yards across, and the ford looked nasty, but the water was gaining in depth and strength every minute, so I had to risk it, and there was no time to test it. I urged my bronco, Chum, through the shallows into the main current. There, where I found the full course of the current mounting up against my horse, my heart turned over with fear. I knew that if Chum's legs were torn from under him I was a dead doctor. Swimming would not save me, for these mountain streams when in flood pound and roll a man under and against the rocks, tear his clothes off and rasp the flesh off his bones. I was dizzy and sick with the swirl and twist of the angry water so near my eyes. The banks seemed to be racing upstream like express trains. I felt the heave of the strong shoulders under me, as my horse strained every nerve.

The water splashed over my saddle horn, and I gave myself up for lost. I let go the reins, grasped the mane of my horse, and sat paralyzed with fear, all my little hope for life in the animal under me. I had often crossed streams on horseback, but never had I been in such danger before. All I could do was to watch with tense nerves the intelligent action of my horse as inch by inch he slowly pushed his body against the current; and even in my fear I was lost in wonder at the skill with which he turned his shoulder to the heavy rushes, felt with his feet for holes or hidden rocks, and with what keen judgment he took advantage of every slack in the current, always calm amid the roaring and splashing, never losing his sense of direction, but keeping to the narrow path of the ford, now covered with deep, tumbling water, as if some uncanny sense guided him, until finally he reached the shallows on the other side, his muscles quivering with the struggle. And yet, such was the spirit of the animal that, after reaching dry ground, he shook himself like a dog, and at once impatiently pulled at the bit, eager to be off on the trail once more.

It was far different with me. I was all in and shaking with nerves. I got off and poured the water out of my boots. I was wet to my cartridge belt. I then rested a bit, sitting on a bank, and let Chum eat a little grass, and when I patted his wet neck and called him a good horse, I could not help thinking that I had played but a sorry part in the crossing of that ford. Here I was a man, supposed to be superior to the beast, and yet, but a few moments before I had been clinging in fear to the hair of that brute, quite helpless, and trusting entirely to this despised brute reason or instinct.

I could not help wondering and thinking over the course of events that gave this bronco of mine such wise and specialized instinct; how in the distant past the Spaniards had lost some of the horses they had brought from Spain; how the strays had then reverted to the wild type on our prairies, and these had grown smaller but tougher, wilder, but more cunning in the years of battling with starvation, wolves, and thirst. The fleetest and most intelligent had survived, and in due course my bronco was born with all the stored wisdom from his forebears, to act promptly in danger, and to have a body and brain trained to survive the dangers of the wilderness.

Lost in these reflections, I suddenly remembered my pack horse, Funny. Upon looking about I could see no trace of him. Had he gone back at the ford? Then I glanced along the surface of the rushing river and, for an instant, I caught a glimpse of four small legs rolling up in the sunlight and then sinking again in the flood. As the river raced around a bend below, I mounted at once and ran my horse along the bank, but the ground was broken, the undergrowth thick, and I felt it was useless. Then I heard my dog Czar barking, and soon I saw him on the bank and there, across the river, was Funny, as naked as when he was born, wet as a drowned rat, calmly eating grass and swishing his tail at the flies as if nothing had happened. I was glad to see him alive, but my pack! All my carefully prepared outfit, my medicine, my surgical kit, my bedroll, all gone for good in that flood and, no doubt, now being carried to the Gulf of Mexico. It was no use worrying; Funny had no doubt kicked himself loose when he was swept off his legs as he followed me at the ford; so I turned east and took the long hot trail into the desert to find Frank, my patient, hidden somewhere in the mass of gulches, buttes, and rocky wastes which were quivering in the heat that stretched for miles before me.

The sun was like fire as it poured down upon us, and hot waves as from a furnace came up from the ground at every step. I was anxious about my Czar—a husky used to snow and ice—and I watched him with some concern as, with flanks heaving and tongue out, he panted his way from one clump of sage to another, flinging himself down in the meager shade they cast, as if at the limit of his strength. Fortunately I had filled my water bag at the river and shared a little water with him from time to time, or, I feel sure, he would have died on the trail. My wet clothes were as dry as tinder in an hour, and the sun was so hot that I was at times dizzy and uncertain of myself. Fortunately I could not lose my way, for the snow mountains far away on the horizon were a sure guide. But I was not so sure of finding the little camp I sought among the sand dunes, dry canyons, and broken surface around me. As the hours passed and we were all becoming worn down by the heat and the blinding light from the alkali plains, I would climb a butte and search every hollow to find the looked-for camp.

At last, to my relief, I saw a few dark specks at the base of a sand hill, quivering and uncertain in the dust and heat waves, and, pushing on, I soon saw a few horses. A man from a group around a blanket tent waved his hat. I was greeted with a hearty welcome, my saddle was taken off, and I was soon by the side of Frank Scott. There he lay on a few saddle blankets, a blanket held over him by rifles stuck in the sand, while thousands of flies covered him. One of the boys was sitting at his head beating them off with his big hat. A sorry sight was poor Frank, warm and dirty from a ten-day drive after cattle in dust and heat. He was shot down just as he was, a stubble of beard on his face, his eyes sunken and his tanned face gone a sickly yellow from pain and loss of blood. But he was game and called out in a cheerful way, "Hello, Doc! Nice hospital this, plenty of sun and air!"

Frank was an old friend of mine, for the year before he had had his thumb caught in the rope against the saddle horn as he roped a steer, and I saw a good deal of him while treating his thumb at that time. He was a good cattleman, knew his business from the ground up; a fine strong young fellow, with light hair, and laughing blue eyes, always joking and a great favorite with all. He was not exactly a model of virtue, for he drank and gambled, as most of the boys did when in town for a good time, but, in a tight place, you could always be sure of Frank.

Reckless and daring, he was true to his code, so I was sorry to see him in such condition. I hated to work on him without ether, but I gave him a shot of morphia in the arm, and a drink of whisky. I found a bit of soap and, with a little water from my water bottle, washed my hands in my turned-up Stetson hat.

Rough Surgery

I cut his shirt away and found a .45 bullet had smashed two ribs on the right side, but had not entered the lung. I got some of the broken bone out and tied a few bleeding places, one of the boys on each arm to keep him quiet. He coughed a lot, the flies settled in droves, the dust blew into the wound, and in the midst of the work, one of the boys fainted and let go of one arm. I had only scissors, one artery forceps, and a scalpel—all I had in my pocket case, whisky and water the only antiseptic.

Another bullet had gone through his right leg below the knee, breaking the big bone rather badly. The temperature in the desert must have been at 120° Fahrenheit, and when I got through with my job, I was about as weak as Frank. The boys were, as usual, as kind and gentle with Frank as any woman could have been. Of course they laughed and joked, and a tenderfoot, looking on, would no doubt have thought them heartless, but nothing could have been further from the truth. These rough men took the ills of life with a laughing gallantry. It was their code never to squeal at fate, but under this reckless manner beat a heart as kind as a child's.

Now I had time to rest, and Frank, after his suffering at my hand, had dropped into a sleep. I could but note the system and energy with which my cowboy friends had acted. After Frank was found wounded, knowing that the nights were as cold as the days were hot in these bad lands, two men had at once ridden off many miles to cut and carry in some firewood, and would be back some time that night. Sandy, as I have told, started off for me, and would return with some food and a bedroll. The others had rigged up a blanket to shelter Frank from the sun, and one had gone out, and after a long search found a crippled calf, shot it, and brought in some meat. It had been decided that all the horses should be driven that night to the river, watered, and allowed to graze in the cool of night, and returned the next morning. Not bad as an example of cowboy headwork, when one considers the difficult situation, miles from wood, water, or grass, and a helpless man too ill to be carried.

At sundown, the boys left with the horses. Frank was still sleeping. It grew dark, and then colder and colder, as the keen night wind came up, so that I was chilled through, and I longed for a fire for warmth and light. It seemed hours that I shivered and walked about to keep warm. Then I heard the boys coming in with the wood, and in no time a cheerful blaze from a campfire lit up the camp, and we were cooking some meat, when along came Sandy with food, bedroll, and five water bags full of water. Sandy said the river was going down, but he had a hard time going across the ford, and had to carry the bedroll on his shoulders to keep it dry. We were now quite jolly, cooking and eating. We lifted Frank onto the mattress and blankets, making him more comfortable, and he then told us the story of the shooting.

We were a rough-looking lot as we sat by Frank's bed. The men had been driving cattle across country for a week or more in a cloud of dust, and were trail dirty, with a stubble of beard and sunburnt faces. As they lounged against their saddles in the glow of the firelight, their big hats pushed back, in high-heeled boots and chaps, every man with his revolver and Winchester ready in a moment for any violent action, they certainly looked the stage bandit. Every face was intent on Frank's story with its tale of treachery so unusual even among these hardened men. No one but Frank spoke; the silence was broken only by Frank's low tones, often interrupted by his cough, the snap of sticks on the fire, and, at times, the howling and yelping of coyotes over the hill, now busy tearing to pieces Frank's dead horse. The night wind, so cold after the heat, moaned faintly among the buttes, and the stars overhead were like diamonds in the clear desert air.

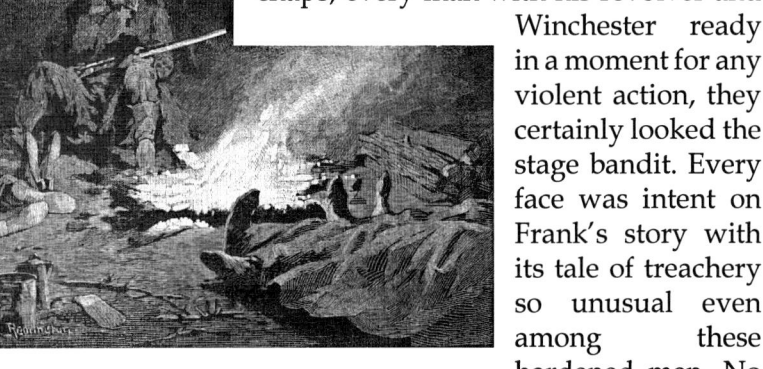

Rough Surgery

The A-Bar-A outfit had driven a big bunch of cattle over this part of the desert, making a short cut to the river. The main herd had gone on, but seven or eight of the boys had stayed to comb up the strays left from the main herd. They made a dry camp and were in the saddle at dawn. Frank was the first to get away, but the others came on a lone steer, could not see his brand, and had to rope him to make sure. This delay saved Frank's life, as they were near enough to hear the shots and to find him after a little search. Riding off by himself and looking all around for cattle, Frank saw a man driving three steers. Frank rode over, as the man did not belong to his crowd. Frank, always reckless, should have known better, for he knew there were some rustlers on the range, but he boldly rode up to the man and found that he was a fellow whom he knew, named Bob Kelly.

Now Kelly had a bad reputation and was suspected of working for some cattle thieves down south, but it was only talk and nothing proved; and when Kelly said, "Hello, Frank," it seemed all right. Frank asked him whose cattle he was driving, and Kelly replied, "Go see for yourself." So Frank rode over to one of the steers with Kelly beside him. Frank tried to see the brand, but it was covered with dust and hard to make out; also, the steer was jumpy and kept sidling away. At this Kelly seemed amused and kept joking Frank. At last Frank got close enough and, bending over to see better, he made out the A-Bar-A on the flank! And that settled it! He knew that the smiling man by him was a rustler stealing cattle from the A-Bar-A.

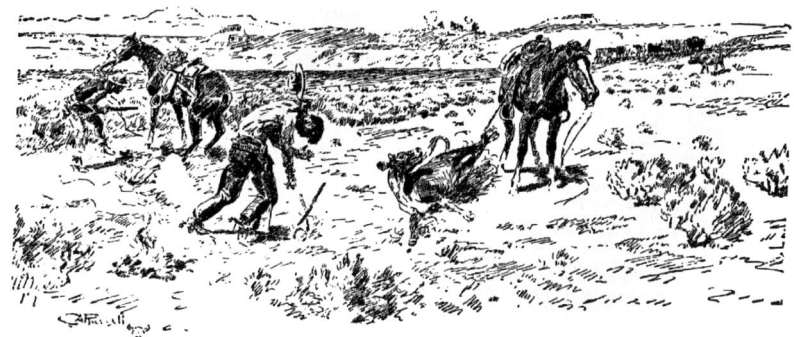

As Frank was swinging back into his saddle and reaching for his gun, there was the bang of a .45, and he felt a blow on his side, as the bullet ripped through his ribs, that nearly threw him off the horse, and then, another bang! and a blow in his leg. His horse gave a jump, staggered a few feet, and, with a shudder and groan, fell crashing to the ground on Frank's leg. He could not move, he felt the blood running down from his side, and pressed his arm tight against it to stop the bleeding. Everything went black as night. He heard the gallop of a horse growing fainter and fainter as Kelly made off at top speed. Then he came to and heard a voice calling out, "Frank!" He tried to call out, but his mouth was full of sand, and he coughed. Then he felt water in his mouth, and one of the A-Bar-A men was holding his head. The man tried to pull him from under his dead horse, but it was too much weight to move; then the man roped one hind leg of the horse, and mounting his bronco, snaked the body free from Frank. Soon the boys came up and all carried him to a better place.

Some of the boys were for following Kelly back, but it was like finding a needle in a haystack, in the country all cut up into canyons and no trail to follow over the stony stretches, so they gave it up and felt that anyway they should stay to help Frank. Of course, Kelly tried to kill Frank to save his own skin, for he knew that the A-Bar-A men were not far off, and that Frank had seen the A-Bar-A brand on the steer, and his only chance was to stop Frank's talking.

We camped in that oven of a desert two days and then packed Frank out on a travois behind a gentle horse, and at last, by short stages, we got him to town. The leg gave some trouble, but finally he recovered and was riding again.

You can be sure he hunted all over for the ranger Kelly, but that rustler escaped to Old Mexico and never came back.

Chapter 12
Coyote Basin

Some of the worst trips that I ever had to make were those across Coyote Basin. This was some miles west of our town, and extended some one hundred miles north and south and fifty miles east and west. This basin was about one hundred feet lower than the country around it and, except for a small spring in the middle, there was no water to be found in the entire region. It was a desert without grass or trees, where the only growing things one could see were cacti, greasewood, and sage bushes, the only signs of life, horned toads, coyotes, and rattlesnakes. If this desert had been a level stretch, crossing it on horseback would have been fairly safe, but the region was a confused mass of rocky buttes, huge boulders, deep sand, with a maze of deep canyons cutting across the trail. The box canyons were from sixty to one hundred feet deep, with walls as straight as a row of house fronts, and the only way to cross them was to find some place where the walls had broken down sufficiently to make it just possible to climb in and out.

Such a country can be crossed only by the bronco, a cow pony trained from birth to such work, and the speed has to be that of a walk, so that a man on horseback, in crossing the basin, will be in luck if, starting at sunrise, he makes the spring in the middle before dark. If lost in this region you are in a bad way, and you die of thirst, so faint and uncertain is the trail across. When at all possible, Indians and cowboys avoid this trail, and weeks pass when no one travels it. Horse thieves made this region a hide-out at times, and one went armed as a matter of course, for these reckless men at that date shot without any warning all who crossed their path.

In winter, crossing the basin was not so dangerous, for the cold air did not worry a horse so much and they stood the thirst better, but in summer, this whole region was like a furnace, the temperature reaching 120° Fahrenheit in the shade, and only a tough pony could go all day without water. There were a few ranches on the other side of the basin from my place, and I often hoped they would keep well and not call me, for I certainly did not fancy any such trip as crossing this beastly desert, while to go around the parched area was a tedious trip of four days at least.

On these long and lonely trips to see a sick or injured ranchman, I had to have a number of horses to ride. These were the small and active broncos used in driving cattle on the range, and my friends, the cowboys, were most kind in buying special ones for my use. At that time I had a string of seven in my corral. I took much time and trouble in training these cow ponies so they would carry me safely over very rough and dangerous trails, not kick me when I put on a horseshoe, or was thrown under their hoofs. They would come to me when called, stand still to be shot over, and allow me to hold on to their tails in climbing a steep trail.

I was the butt of many jokes, and the boys called my corral the "circus" from the queer doings that went on there during my horse training; but it paid, for I could always rely on my horse friends in a tight place.

On August 2, 1884, I had been in such pain from a sick headache that I could not sleep. Now a sick headache is only a minor illness, but if you have the regular old-fashioned variety, it is no light affair. I inherited mine from three generations; every three weeks I had to suffer intense pain in the head for twenty-four hours, ending with vomiting and weakness. On this occasion I was having a bad one, and just before dawn I heard a horse coming at a lope. Outside my open window it stopped, and a voice called out, "Oh, Doc!"

I knew the voice. It was a cowboy called Jim, from the L. O. T. Ranch. I crawled to my window and leaned out. I could just make out the shadow of a man and horse near my fence.

"Yes, Jim!" I called, "what's the matter?"

"Well, Doc," said Jim, "word came to us at the ranch that Bill Dern on the other side of the basin had been throwed and drug among stumps, has a broken leg, and near dead, and they want you."

Here was a nice outlook! I was so sick I could hardly stand, and I must ride two days across that hell of a Coyote Basin in August. I could not take a pack horse with some comforts. With all those rattlesnakes I did not wish to risk my dogs' being bitten. I had to go light to make time. I am ashamed to say I was tempted to back out. I told myself I was too ill to face such a trip in the heat; it was no use killing myself for these people; but this lasted only for a moment, and I called out to Jim to get Buck out of the corral and saddle him while I dressed. Buck was a yellow buckskin-colored bronco, not pretty to look at, but one of the best I had on a rough trail, and he was shod, while the others were bare.

I was dressed in no time, filled my canteen, got some chocolate bars, and half a dozen meat sandwiches. Jim had Buck at the door, with saddlebags all in place. I gave a glance at my soft bed, so quiet and restful to my pain and weakness, and with an "All right, Jim," I closed the door and mounted Buck. As usual he was a bit frisky. I suppose the cool air of the dawn, a tight cinch, and a bronco's sense of humor inspired him, because he gave a few stiff-legged crow hops to show me he could buck if he wanted to, and made my head ache with the jolting.

Then we were on our way. The town was dark and silent, and in an hour I was at the edge of Coyote Basin and looking down at the weird scene as the sun rose. I felt so ill I got off Buck and threw myself under a piñon tree. Here I had a nervous chill, an attack of vomiting, and had to struggle with the idea of giving up, but I felt I must go on. A loss of self-respect was worse than anything the desert could do to me, so I rode Buck down the steep trail into the basin. It grew hotter every step, and when the sun got up overhead it burned my back through my shirt like a fire, and my rifle barrel was too hot to touch. I rode in a kind of stupor. What with the heat and the glare from the sand and rocks, my head was so bad that I did not care what happened.

About noon I felt my sick headache was getting better. I could not eat yet, but I drew in under the shade of a rock, got off, and examined Buck's shoes, for a cast shoe meant a lame horse and my finish. I took a small drink of the water in the canteen; every drop was precious; as I corked the canteen, Buck's keen ears caught the gurgle of water, and he turned his head and looked into my face with such a look of reproach, or what my guilty conscience took to be reproach, that I was ashamed of myself. He was awfully thirsty, the poor brute, so I soaked up a handkerchief in the precious water, held Buck's head up, and squeezed the water from the handkerchief on the back of his dry tongue. It was only a drop to him, of course, but it refreshed him a bit anyhow.

We were following the trail through a weird and strange formation of red sandstone, in huge buttes and spires, unnatural forms like animals, or human figures, and as the trail wound in and out among these fantastic shapes and the heat waves made them seem to dance before my eyes, I felt I was having some dreadful nightmare. There was not a breath of air, and the heat from the rocks as I passed by them hit me like a blow.

We came suddenly on the canyons and gulches crossing the deep trail, deep and of appalling steepness, so that it seemed impossible for any horse to carry a man in and out. As I rode up

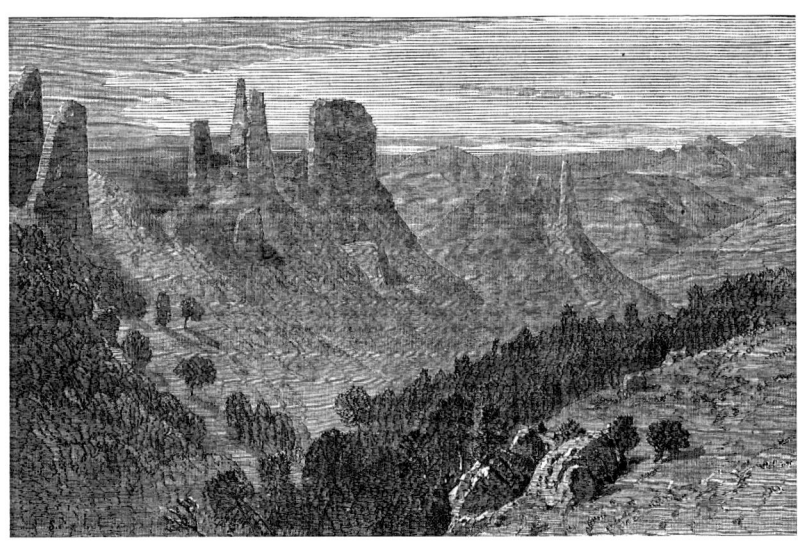

to the edge of the first one and looked down the almost straight face to the narrow floor so far below me, I felt my heart racing in fear.

There was nothing to do. I had to go on. I was still too weak to dismount and climb, and I knew my horse Buck was far too good a cow pony to need any hints or control from me, so I gave him his head and, leaning far back in the saddle and clutching the back cinch near the saddle, gave myself up to Buck and fate. I still had some curiosity to see how Buck would manage it, and I soon had the opportunity. Buck let his front feet slip over the edge, drew his hind feet under him, and in a moment we were sliding down. Every now and then when we were going too fast I could feel Buck making frantic digs with his hind feet to hold us. I felt that he must be standing on his head; and then, with a rattle of stones and a dense cloud of dust, we were on the soft sand at the bottom. I had no time to think, for Buck, with a glance at the wall above us, commenced to climb up.

I fear I was a comic figure of a horseman on that ascent as, with arms clasped around my horse's neck, I clung desperately as Buck, in a series of buck jumps, made his way upward. I could hear the stones go bounding down behind us, and feel Buck struggle for breath until finally we were on top, Buck drenched in sweat, trembling from the exertion, and his breath coming in gasps. I let out his cinches—I used two on my saddle in hilly country—to give him his wind, and on we went, climbing in and out of those infernal canyons until I thought they would never end.

And then when we came to the last of them, and they were not so steep, but easier to cross, we had a tumble. Perhaps we were both careless, or the ground was softer; anyway, we had crossed a small one and had nearly reached the top on the other side when, as Buck gave a last heave to reach the level ground, I felt him slowly sinking under me as the whole bank crumbled with us. At first we sank down so gently I tried to swing free, but my foot caught in my slicker roll back of the saddle and in a moment I felt myself turning over and over. I was so confused by the dust that blinded and choked me, and the rattle of stones sliding down with us, that I did not know what had happened until with a thump we landed at the bottom. I lay on my side, my left leg under Buck, who was kicking and making frantic efforts to get up. Every time he moved he hurt my leg so badly that I was growing faint with the pain. I reached over and slapped Buck's side and yelled out for him to stop. He understood me. I had trained him for just such a mishap and, like the good pony he was, he stopped struggling.

Fortunately the sand was deep and soft under us, and I dug the sand away under my leg so I could drag it out from the weight on it. As soon as I was loose Buck got up and shook the sand from him like a wet dog. I anxiously examined my leg. It was bruised and the skin scraped off in places, but I was thankful no bones were broken, and in five minutes I could walk on it, though with some pain and a bad limp. I was a bit nervous after the fall. I took a drink of whisky out of my medical kit and, fearing to ride up that hill, I made Buck go first and, holding onto his tail, I was able to limp up the hill to the top. At last those dreadful canyons were passed, and our trail was fairly level, deep in sand, and heavy going, but no climbing. Buck made hardly any noise as we trotted along this sand trail, and I suppose we were both rather stupid in the heat and silence.

I had heard some rather wild stories about the rattlesnakes in the basin and, as I had seen none so far in the trip, heard not even a rattle, I decided that the boys had been trying to scare me. I realized later that only in certain places in the basin were there so many. I must have entered one of these snake zones because, as we jogged along with all quiet and peaceful, Buck gave a snort of fear and made a jump to one side of the trail. He stood trembling and looking back to see what had scared him, and so I saw a big old rattlesnake right in the middle of the trail, all coiled up, his tail up in the air rattling like mad. Now, I have no horror of snakes. I am used to them, and have caught them alive, killed them, and cut them up, but I also am very careful not to risk any chance of being bitten by one, and I always kill one when I can. They are a danger to be feared and avoided. I dismounted and walked up to within ten feet of this big fellow on the trail, took careful aim with my Colt, and let him have it in the middle of the big ring of coils. My gun sounded like a cannon in the silence, then through a cloud of dust and smoke, I caught a glimpse of his body as, nearly cut in two, it was thrown up into the air, twisting and turning, his yellow belly shining in the sun. I rode on now, watching every foot of the trail ahead. In the next four miles I shot five more, all in the trail, and then I saw no more. I heard some rattling as I passed along, but I was in a hurry and had no time for killing snakes on the side of the trail.

It must have been late in the day, for the sun was getting lower, when ahead of us I saw a low flat valley covered with what looked like a snow field so white and sparkling in the sunshine as almost to blind one. I knew from what I had been told that this was an old lake bed covered with alkali. As we rode over this white plain, Buck's hoofs broke through a thin crust; a dense white cloud of fine alkali dust rose around us, and in no time we were covered as if with flour. It smarted our eyes and set us both coughing. I did not care; I knew that Rattlesnake Joe's place with the only water was near the other edge of this old lake bed, and as we passed over a ridge I could see, in a little gulch, a shack made of poles, a small corral and two burros inside, and I knew that this place was the halfway station where I could give my horse water and stay for the night.

I looked around the gulch where Joe had his home and saw nothing but the arid sand hills, a lonely, miserable place. The little shack, made of sticks and mud, with dirt for a roof, half buried in the bank, was so crude and primitive it seemed a poor shelter for a dog. I noticed smoke coming out of a pipe in the roof. No signs, no dogs, only the burros standing motionless in the corral. I rode a little nearer, and from behind the shelter of a sandbank watched the hut. The door was shut. I remembered all the strange tales I had heard of this strange man, called by the cattlemen "Rattlesnake Joe"; how he was a tough customer, about fifty years old, was known to have served a term in prison, was suspected of selling whisky to the Indians. All agreed that he was half-crazy and had a lot of rattlesnakes as pets, so they gave him his name.

I was curious to see this grim hermit, but was rather nervous about it. I suspect I was foolish, but I pulled my rifle out from its sheath under my left leg and carried it across the horn of my saddle; I wanted to be ready for anything this crazy man might do. I drew up about fifty yards from the cabin, and cried out, "Oh, Joe!" I called several times—utter silence. Then a small shutter was thrown back, a rifle barrel thrust out aimed at me, and a shrill voice cried out, "Who the hell are you?" Now I was not scared by this. If this man had intended to shoot he would have done so before. I told him who I was and where I was going. The rifle was pulled in, the door opened, and the hermit, unarmed, stood in the sand outside calling to me, "Come on, Doc. It's all right." I rode right up to him, and he said with a laugh, "Sorry I held you up, but the rustlers are all about the basin and I have to be careful." I looked with some interest at this strange specimen of humanity: a small, wiry man of middle age, tanned dark as an Indian, small, cunning eyes, his hair falling on his shoulders, a ragged beard, so dirty and unwashed as to be repulsive. He wore an old red shirt, a filthy pair of buckskin trousers; his bare feet scratched up the sand with the toes of one foot as he talked. He was a crafty liar, a shifty old jailbird, with deceit written all over him.

I must make the best of it, for I had to have water and rest, so I was all smiles, and lay myself out to be as friendly as I could. I watched him pretty closely all the same. He was sane enough, led me to the spring, only a faint trickle, but caught in a barrel it gave Buck a good drink. Joe led me to the hut and motioned me to go in. I had forgotten all about the snake stories and I bent down and stood in the low doorway. It looked more like a wolf's den than a cabin: two bunks, a table, boxes as chairs, a litter of old skins, rope, cooking pots and pans, some pack saddles—all black with smoke. The floor was made of poles laid close together, and not of earth as was usual. I knew there must be some kind of cellar under this pole floor and wondered what on earth this man could do with a cellar under such a shack of sticks and mud.

I took a step or so, and the whole floor bent under my weight. Poles rolled together, making a clatter, and above this sound, keen and shrill, a sinister warning to man and beast, arose a chorus of rattling so penetrating and intense that in the small room it seemed to me that a hundred rattlesnakes were all around me. I fancied I could see them in the cabin interior, hanging down from the roof and walls. I was so badly scared that in a panic I turned and dashed for the door, running full tilt into Joe coming in with a bucket of water.

The impact carried us through the doorway; we fell outside locked together in a wild scramble. The water was spilled over us. We sprang up in a moment, my fear turned to anger, and I gave Joe a tongue-lashing. That old reprobate took it fairly well. I suppose he felt guilty and realized what a scare I had had. Anyway he told me that his pet rattlesnakes were in a cellar under the cabin, that they could not climb up to the floor or get out, and he said he forgot to warn me that there was no danger and all their rattling was because they were afraid. He was anxious, he said, to "tote" one up on a stick and show me how tame and harmless they were. I fear I was a bit too quick in my declining this free show, and his feelings were hurt.

Joe cooked the usual mess called food on the frontier; coffee, biscuits, beans, and bacon; then, over a pipe after dinner he grew quite confidential about his rattlesnakes. He told me as a great secret that he was fond of snakes, had learned to tame them from the Indians down in Arizona and New Mexico, and his one ambition in life was to train a few of his "pets," take them to some town, and join some show as a snake charmer—a practical idea, and one in which he was successful sometime later, as I afterward heard.

I confess, I looked this dirty cabin over with some suspicion before going to bed in my bunk, but was firmly assured by Joe's saying, "Why, Doc, I wouldn't have you bit in my cabin for a farm." So I tumbled in, so tired that I slept soundly and was called by Joe at sunup. More coffee and bacon, and I found Buck in the corral. A loose shoe was nailed fast, saddle put on, canteen filled, and just as the sun came over a ridge I called "So long" to Joe and soon was out on the desert again, glad to be in clean air and away from the smells and dirt of the vile cabin, not to mention the crazy man and his queer "pets."

The trail was fairly easy now, some deep sand, but my good horse kept up his easy fox trot, mile after mile. The heat was something awful, but I was growing hardened to it. I saw no living thing all day, just the desert and a blazing sun in the silence. It must have been the middle of the afternoon when, far ahead, I saw a horse. Now a horse in this desert might mean anything, most likely horse thieves. I kept behind rocks and sand hills, with rifle ready, and at every ridge I looked over the country carefully. Nothing else was in sight, and at last I was near enough to see the horse plainly. He stood like a stone horse, never moving. His head looked strange, too big for his body. I now rode up close. He was a cow pony, standing with legs far apart as if afraid of falling. His head was so swollen that he could just breathe, making a horrible kind of whistle. Covered with sweat, with flanks heaving, and his legs trembling under him, he was a sad sight. He wore no saddle or bridle. I could see he was near the end, yet I knew I must not shoot him for you did not meddle with stray horses on the range in those days. Of course, I knew that he was suffering from snake bite and I could visualize the tragic little history of this cow pony easily enough. As a stray from the horse herd of some cow outfit, he had wandered into the basin and, traveling along with head low, looking for grass, he had bumped into a big rattler on the trail. He had been struck on the nose, and the poison had rapidly extended, and now he was beyond help. I longed to shoot him, but did not dare, and so with a sad heart I rode off, the gasping of his choking breath following me for a long time.

At last we commenced to go up a steep hill, and I knew we were leaving the basin, and as we rode over a little divide we saw some timber ahead and then, here and there, a patch of buffalo grass. Soon we were in among a grove of cottonwoods. Never had the shade of green leaves seemed more wonderful to me after the glare of yellow sand and rocks baking under the fierce rays of the sun. It was a change so sudden as to seem like some enchantment to my eyes, so long dazzled by the blinding light of the desert.

I knew I was approaching my goal, and Buck sensed the nearness of water. As he quickened his trot we at last passed over a low divide, and through the timber I caught a glimpse of a green valley with a stream wandering down amid groves of cottonwoods, a fenced field with horses grazing, a big corral, and a house with a real shingle roof, glass windows, and a bit of garden fenced and trees before it. I rode down the trail and soon was near enough to see a woman come running out of the house, followed by three small children and a sheep dog. All stood at the garden gate, the woman

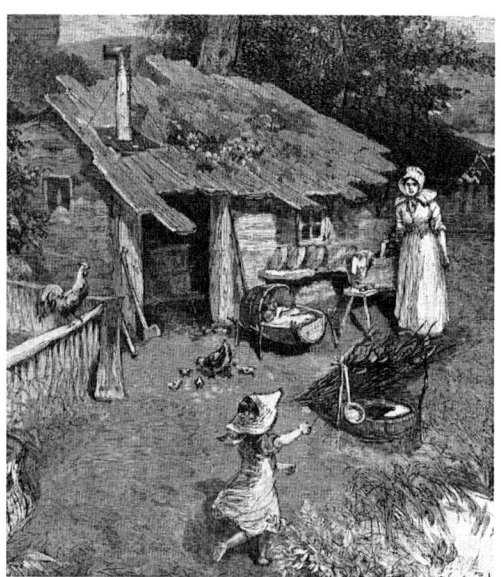

shielding her eyes with her hand and looking anxiously towards me. I rode up close and, as the woman ran out to meet me, she managed to gasp, "Oh, Doctor, I thought you would never come! Will is *so* bad!" And leaning against my horse, she sobbed and cried for a bit, and then urged me to come and see her husband. This was, I knew, Mrs. Dern, a fine type of ranchwoman, about thirty-five, strong and capable. The poor woman had been all alone, with her husband badly injured, three children to care for, cooking and nursing for five days of anxiety. No wonder she looked worn out.

I turned Buck out, took my saddlebags, and went into the house. It was as clean and neat as it could be—four rooms and plain furniture. I found Will Dern on the bed. He looked bad, his tan a dirty yellow, his cheeks and eyes sunken; a big man, he had wasted away to a shadow. He could only whisper, but with the true cowboy courage he smiled and said, "Hello, Doc!"

I stripped him; his left leg was drawn up, and I found it dislocated, the hipbone out of the socket, his left arm and side badly bruised and cut. I knew I could never get the hip back by main force. It was necessary to relax the muscles first. So, to make him unconscious, I poured some chloroform on a towel and told Mrs. Dern how to hold it over Bill's face. Mrs. Dern was fine and did as I told her. When he was well under, I turned the leg up, and pulled it around so that at last, after three or four attempts, it snapped into its socket again. I was quite happy. I had feared it was broken at first, but just as I was congratulating myself on my successful operation we had a little mix-up that was a curious performance. Mrs. Dern, worn out by the strain and chloroform vapor, suddenly fainted and fell on the floor; the children, huddled in a corner, let out a series of yells; and as I bent over Mrs. Dern to put a wet handkerchief on her face, the shepherd dog, thinking I was the villain of the play and killing the family, rushed at me and gave me a hard bite on that portion of my body that was very tender from hard riding.

However, the confusion was soon over. Mrs. Dern got up and insisted on cooking supper. Bill came out of his chloroform jag and said his leg hurt awful, but was in place, he felt. The children were bundled outside to play; the dog saw his mistake; while I sat in a rocker smoking a cigarette and watching the skillful hands of Mrs. Dern as she fried bacon, made hot biscuits, and brewed strong coffee.

I had three restful days at the Dern ranch, just loafed about, played with the children, and enjoyed the company of these simple, fine people. Bill Dern recovered in a wonderful way. I rubbed his stiff leg, and dressed his battered arm.

He had, he told me, been thrown from a wild bronco he was "aiming to gentle." His foot had caught in the stirrup as he was thrown, and he had been dragged over the ground among stones and stumps of trees until the cinch of the saddle broke, and the saddle fell off—a very close call for him. Mrs. Dern had seen the whole thing and had rushed out and carried her husband to the cabin. She was a very strong woman, and the distance was only a few feet; still it was a wonder. Love and excitement had given her abnormal strength.

On the third day a young fellow, Charlie Dern, a cousin of Bill, came riding in from a ranch some fifty miles south; he had heard of the accident only that day. So I left this little family in good hands and rode around the basin to reach home. I could not face another night at Rattlesnake Joe's shack, or the heat of the desert. It took me four days, but the trail was good. I made a ranch every night and did a bit of doctoring on the way—all small stuff—pulled a couple of bad teeth, got a piece of steel out of an eye, and at another ranch made a truss out of leather for an old rupture. It paid my way, fed my horse, and made friends.

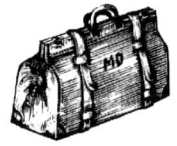

Chapter 13
A Storm Baby

Some of the settlers that came in were a curious lot—often with only a few cows. They built rough shacks and took up the land where there was some natural pasture, and, living from hand to mouth, hoped for the day when they could sell out and move on. Many of them were shiftless and lazy, not able to make a living, so they led a miserable existence in leaky, cold cabins, with dirt everywhere and harsh, wild nature to battle with to keep body and soul together. Ranches were few and far between, for people as yet were widely scattered over this region.

Not all of our settlers were of the nondescript kind I have described; some of them were of quite another type: good reliable cattlemen in a small way, who took up a ranch or, more often, bought out a settler for a small sum. John Good and his wife were of this better class. They were both young, Jack thirty and his wife twenty. From an old pioneer family near Denver, they were people of education and knew how to manage. They brought in about a hundred head of stock, turned most of it out on the open range, keeping only two or three cows to milk and a few horses to ride. They settled in a wild country in a little valley eighteen miles away from my town, their nearest neighbors being in the town.

They were used to the life and had some means to live on. Jack built a regular old-fashioned cabin of big logs, well chinked, a dirt roof, and a plank floor, making a big room about eighteen by twenty. Then they had to furnish the cabin, and that was a task—to pack things over the trail. Mrs. Good insisted upon having carried in the big bed she was born in, which was given her by her mother. It was a huge affair made of walnut, with a feather bed, big enough for a family to sleep in; and when at last

A Storm Baby

in place, although scarred and scratched by the bushes as it was packed in on horses, it was the wonder of all who saw it. With a few chairs and a table, and with the cookstove glowing, it was a cozy place when all was settled. I remember there were curtains at the windows, and a box of red geraniums—all very cozy and homelike to see in that wild place.

Jack Good was a big strong man, a hard worker, and skillful with ax or rifle. He was a favorite with all, and so jolly it made one laugh to see his big red face and blond beard, his blue eyes always dancing with fun and good humor. When he heard a joke you could hear him laugh a mile away. Anne, his wife, was another of the same kind. Strong and straight, with her hair in a long pigtail down her back, a poke bonnet, and gingham dress and apron, with red arms showing to the elbows, she would not be considered exactly stylish today; but she was so sweet and natural, so strong and capable, that she seemed born to be a good wife to a wilderness breaker. Nothing discouraged her in the least, and when they were living in a tent while building their cabin, I have seen her cooking over an open fire with the rain pouring down, serving a good dinner with a smile on her face and the water slopping over her feet. Jack, of course, adored her, and I often thought how much happier these simple people were in their hard life than many a couple with a fortune.

The Goods had been married for three years and were quite sad over having had no children; so when, one day soon after Christmas, Jack rode in to our place and told me Anne expected a baby in February, I felt as pleased as he did over the news. Jack was anxious to have Anne come in to our little town to be near me and close to some women when the baby came, but Anne would have none of it, and, being a young woman of decided character, of course had her way. She wanted to have her baby in the old bed she was born in, and her married sister was coming from Cheyenne to be with her. Jack was to ride in for me when I was needed, so all was arranged and everything was in order. But Fate came and spoiled our plans.

About a week later, Slim Tex, a rider for the A-Bar-A outfit, came galloping up in a frightful hurry one afternoon and told me that he had been hunting up some strayed stock by Good's ranch. He stopped at the cabin, and Mrs. Good came out and told him that her husband had left early in the morning to be gone two days cutting cedar posts somewhere up in the mountains; that she had been all right until noon, but then she had had a severe pain and had had pain ever since. She was all alone and was sure her baby was coming a month before she expected it. She told Slim to go for me as quickly as he could. Slim could not hunt up Jack in the thick timber. There were no neighbors nearer than town, so he burned the trail up to me. At the news Slim told me I was in such a hurry that I never thought of hunting up some woman in the settlement to go along to help me with Mrs. Good, but in ten minutes I was on the road and pushing my bronco to the limit.

I was worried, thinking of Mrs. Good all alone at such a time, and I felt better when I topped the last rise and, below me in the valley, saw the cabin. In the doorway was Mrs. Good, her hand shading her eyes as anxiously she looked along the trail for me. I gave her a call and waved my hat; she waved back and went into the cabin again. Picking my way down the rough trail, I saw a dark mass of clouds gathering over the hills, and before I reached the cabin it had suddenly grown much colder. Snowflakes as sharp as needles were beating in my face, and I knew we were in for a winter blizzard.

As I entered the cabin I found Mrs. Good on the bed, suffering a hard pain. She just said, "Thank God, you are here, Doctor. Please see about the stock." So I fought my way to the corral, turned my horse loose, forked some hay up in the open shed for the

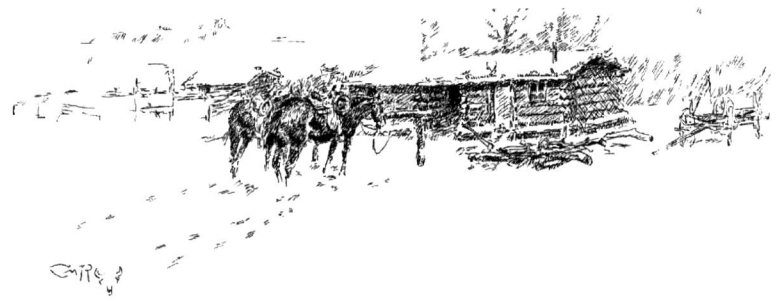

A Storm Baby

stock—some five cows and two horses—and left them all huddled up in one end. It was now storming so fiercely that I could not see a foot into the drift that cut like a knife and blinded me. I fell down and feared to move for a moment; men had been frozen to death in such storms, lost within one hundred feet of their cabins. At last I found a rope stretched from the corral to the house to act as a guide at night, or in a blizzard, and blessed Jack for his good sense in having put it up. I slid my hand along the rope, bumped into the cabin, and at last found the door and burst in, my nose and ears white and one hand frosted. Mrs. Good insisted upon my rubbing snow on my frozen skin.

I found that Jack had enough stovewood cut up to last a week, so we had a good fire and a warm cabin. Mrs. Good felt better and helped me cook some supper, but she could not eat. It was now dark, and we lit candles. I remember we joked about it all and pretended we did not care, for Mrs. Good was worrying about her husband camping out in the storm. I told her he was in the thick timber with blankets and food, wood for a good fire, and that an old-timer such as he was would, I felt sure, be quite safe. She was a good sport, so smiled and tried to be cheerful.

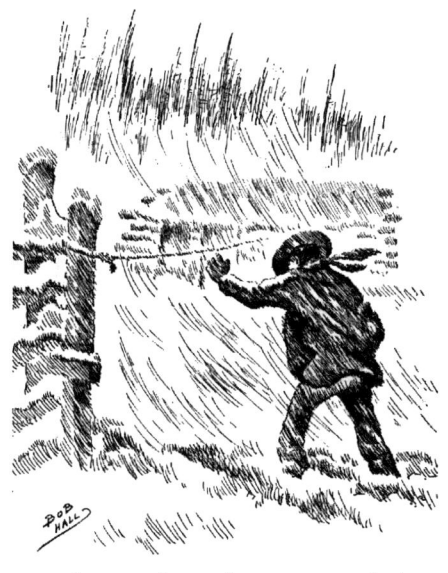

It grew colder and colder, and must have been away below zero, because I noted a thing that never happened unless it was very cold: the big logs of the cabin every now and then snapped like a pistol shot as the frost ate into them. The wind rushed by with a roar like thunder, and we had to shout to be heard. The windows were soon plastered up outside by the snow, and a big drift covered the door. The wind drifted the snow under the door and made a white heap that the stove heat melted, until I stuffed some gunny sacks along the bottom of the door. I got all ready with hot water, and all my instruments under a cloth on the table, washed my hands, and borrowed an apron from Mrs. Good. The hours passed slowly, with poor Mrs. Good suffering intensely, and the wind trying to blow the cabin over. I was thankful as these gusts struck it that it was built so strongly, the big logs all around and the dirt roof weighing tons holding it down like a rock.

As I sat there in that cabin, all alone with my patient, I could not resist a smile at the contrast between my present position and the maternity room of the big hospital where I treated such cases in New York, and, as I watched, by the light of the stove, the little drifts of snow come sifting in through every crack, heard the roar of the wind, and felt the deadly cold increase hour by hour, I pictured that white and spotless delivery room, so warm, so sheltered from any noise or draught; those white-robed nurses, so alert and skilled in their duties; that trained anesthetist, so sure and safe; that chief in charge ready to help a novice over the hard places; all so complete, so restful, that one was merely part of a well-oiled machine, while here I was completely cut off from any help, no matter what happened.

At midnight my patient was growing so weak from pain that I became anxious. She implored me to do something, and, with many misgivings, at last I decided to use instruments. I feared giving chloroform, but it must be done singlehanded or not at all; so I put some cotton in the bottom of a glass tumbler, poured some chloroform on the cotton, and had my patient hold it over her mouth and nose. When she lost consciousness, her hand relaxed, and the tumbler fell off—a dangerous way enough, I knew, for she might get too much. It was nervous work keeping one eye on that tumbler to see that it did fall off before an overdose was taken. I had to put the candle far away for fear of the fumes of chloroform catching fire, and it was so dark that I could not see my patient's face. I could not stop to put on wood, and it grew so cold as the fire died out that I was shaking with cold, my hands were numb, and the forceps like ice.

There seemed to be hours of struggle, but at last that welcome first cry of a newborn baby was heard above the roar of the wind. I made up a big fire, and we were warm again. It was a boy. I must have made an amusing figure as, with one of Mrs. Good's aprons on, I held that youngster in my thin and uncomfortable lap in front of the stove and unskillfully proceeded to wash him. He was as slippery as an eel, squirming every way, red with anger, and yelling his little head off. And the anxious mother calling out from the bed, "Be careful, Doctor, his feet are too near the stove; don't burn him," rattled me so that I hardly knew what I was doing.

I can laugh at it now, but then we were very serious over it. The mother twenty and the serious doctor twenty-six! At last the baby was safe in a little warmed blanket by his mother, and she smiled down at it, that wonderful smile that has greeted so many mortals, all pain forgotten, nothing but pride and joy — an old story, but always new and pure and sweet.

I was suddenly all in, felt faint, and lay down on the cold floor ashamed of my weakness. I hoped Mrs. Good would not notice, but that young mother was all interest in a moment.

"Now, Doctor, don't be silly; you are tired out. Lie down on the bed. I won't have you lying on that cold floor."

I was too sick and cold to care, and it was fine to stretch out on the outside of that big old bed and sink into the soft feathers. I pulled an extra blanket over me. The storm had blown itself out, and the silence was broken only by the cracking of the snow as it settled on the roof. I heard a little cry like the pipe of a bird and knew it was made by the baby, and that all was well, and, tired out, I was soon asleep.

I was awakened by stamping and the scraping of a shovel at the door; someone was digging us out. I heard Jack's deep voice, "Are you all right, Anne?" and Anne called out, "All right, Jack." The door was flung open, and bright sunshine flooded the room. Mrs. Good whispered, "Keep still! I want to surprise him." Then, in came Jack, all covered with snow and, in his fur coat, looking as big as a grizzly bear. He shook himself like a wet dog. When he shut the door the cabin was almost dark, the windows were so banked with snow.

As Jack bent over the bed Anne pulled back the blanket and showed him his son on her arm. Jack was so surprised he could only gasp, "Oh, Anne, were you alone? I never dreamed of this—and you could not send for the doctor?"

Anne smiled and pointed to me on the bed.

This was too much for Jack and, with roars of laughter, he did a sort of war dance around the cabin, shouting out, "Well, I have got one on you, Doc. Wait till I tell the boys how I came home and found you in bed with my wife. What will you say to square it, Doc?"

And then Anne, mad all through, half rose in bed and gave Jack a calling down, saying she would not have her little doctor made a joke of, that he had saved her life and the baby's. Then she broke into tears.

Jack was sober in an instant and down on his knees by the bed, while I got up and put on my boots. Jack was very sorry and said he could not help seeing the funny side of it. At last we all laughed, admired the baby, and soon were cooking flapjacks for breakfast.

Jack had had a hard time of it on his trip. He got to the timber all right, then the blizzard caught him. He made a big fire, cut branches, and built a windbreak, then cooked supper. He was sheltered in the timber, and his horse could stand it in a deep thicket of young pines. Then a queer thing happened to Jack. He was one of the most simple and direct persons I ever knew, a big strong animal with no imagination at all, and what happened to him was so weird that he could not get over the wonder of it. As he sat by that fire in the dark forest with the wind bending the big treetops over his head, and the snow piling up in drifts, he seemed to have a message so real that it struck his mind like a blow. It was a feeling that Anne needed him. He seemed to hear her voice rising above the storm, saying, "Jack! Jack!" He tried to argue himself out of it by thinking: Anne is all right, good cabin, plenty of wood, but no use, the feeling was stronger than reason. He said he knew she wanted him, as plainly as if she had really called him. Half desperate with anxiety, he could do nothing but wait for daylight. He well knew that to attempt to struggle in the dark through that killing cold, and travel over the trail he had come, would mean falling down some cliff or into a canyon; so poor Jack suffered all night, tramping around the fire, and at the first faint light came battling through the drifts. The horse could not travel in the deep snow, so Jack left him, and walked. When he reached the last hill and saw smoke coming from the stovepipe of his home below him in the valley, he knew someone was keeping the fire up; and when he at last reached us and learned what had happened and how Anne, in her pain, had thought of him, his wonder at that voice calling him up there in the woods never ceased.

 The mother and baby being all right, I was anxious to start home, although the Goods were urging me to stay. I had rather a hard trip. I kept to the ridges where the snow was blown off, but often I had to lead my horse where I tramped a trail in the deep snow for him to follow. It was clear and still, with a warm sun, but the plowing along in snow up to my knees in the bad places was exhausting, and I was a wet and tired doctor when at last I reached my own cabin.

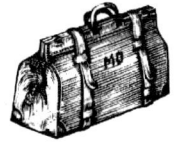

Chapter 14
Mule Surgery

After the snow was gone the town awoke to new life and activity. Huge ore wagons that freighted the crude ore collected by miners during the long winter passed slowly through our main street. These wagons were hauled by teams of mules — not ordinary mules, but splendid, upstanding beasts that were the pride and delight of their owners who, as a rule, treated them with a care and devotion shown only to race horses. Every buckle was shining, red rosettes were on their headstalls, a big scarlet pompon bobbed proudly above their long ears, and a string of silver bells on their collars made music at every step. Their eyes were bright and alert, and their coats shining with the careful grooming, for these teams earned big money in boom silver days, and were not only the pets and companions of their owners, but were a paying investment, and as such were carefully guarded and treated.

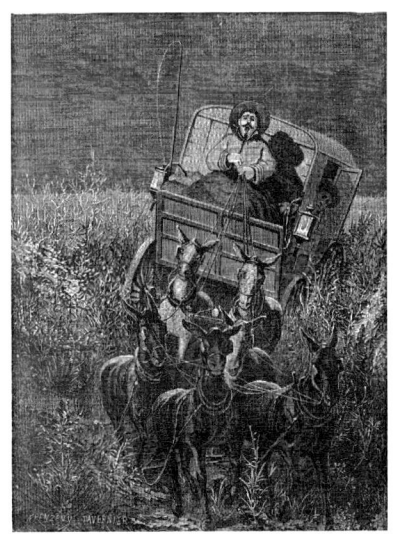

One team of four mules always interested me more than the others that passed before my office because they were in a class by themselves. Splendid animals, of a cream color, they were in top condition, their harness shining and polished, their coats like satin. Powerfully built, they moved with a dignity and grace that told of their strength and breeding, and they obeyed every word of their

Mule Surgery

owner and driver without the need of using the reins at all. In fact, they were known to be the crack team of our camp and the last word in mule perfection. Abe Brown was the owner, and no one could be prouder or fonder of his prize team than Abe, who lavished care and devotion upon them as if they were his children. I came to know Abe by his calling me in to see his daughter, a pretty little thing of five, and not very ill, so she was soon all right; and I won Abe's regard by petting and admiring his mules.

I did not see Abe for two or three weeks, and then one day he appeared at my office with a very long face and told me his trouble. It appeared that one of his beloved mules—the best one of the four, and his leader—had a growth on his shoulder which had gradually grown so large that it hung down, making him limp, and, of course, of no use in harness. Abe used a two-mule team but, of course, this meant half a load, and here in the middle of the summer with everything booming, he was losing money every day. Abe had tried to cure this tumor by blistering and ointments, but it was growing larger; nothing had helped a bit. Abe was desperate, and as a last resort came to me, a doctor of human beings, to ask if I could doctor a mule! As Abe said, "Doc, I know you regular doctors don't fancy doctoring mules none, but I thought you might for once have a go at my mule. You see, having a horse doctor from Denver would cost more than the mule is worth, and then he might know nothing when he got here; some don't." I felt sorry for Abe, but I knew nothing about mules. We do not handle mules in New York, and I was frankly afraid of the beasts, as I remember helping in an operation on a crushed skull one time in the hospital and was told the patient had been kicked by a mule.

So it was with some misgivings that I followed Abe to a stable to see his mule. I saw that Abe was rather scornful at the way I played safe and reached over from an empty stall to make my examination from this safe position, for I had visions of that mule's nearly biting my head off if I hurt him. I was taking no chances. Abe's remark, "Gentle as a kitten, Doc," was quite lost on my timid and skeptical mind. I found a tumor as large as a big watermelon, freely movable, and I told Abe I could cut it out. Abe was much delighted, so the next morning was set for the clinic. In my kit I found a sail needle about six inches long with which I used to sew canvas, and with some big cod lines and a rubber apron I appeared at the corral just out of town, ready for my maiden mule effort.

I did not expect an audience, but to my horror there was quite a crowd gathered; the word had in some way got around, and there on the top rail of the corral were miners, cowboys, barkeeps, and loafers in general, all wearing broad grins and in high good humor, and quite in the spirit of a baseball game. Their sarcastic comments and rough jokes at my expense were greeted by laughter, hoots, and yells. I was nervous enough anyway, and this open-air clinic did not act as a sedative, by any means, but I had to go on. A big pile of straw was heaped in the center of the corral, the poor limping mule was led up to it, and a couple of cowboys in no time had roped and hog-tied that mule "fore and aft" so that he could not move a leg, and even my fear of kicking was set at rest.

Two volunteers sat close by and batted the flies away with their big hats. I was amazed at the size of the beast; he seemed to tower over me as huge as an elephant as he lay there so helpless, his big body heaving up and down with every breath. The restless animal constantly twitched his skin as if flies bit him. The only practical way I could reach the tumor was to sit on the mule's side as if riding him, and at every deep breath he took I was rocked back and forth as if I were on a rocking horse, in, I fear, a most undignified manner. The crowd, at any rate, thought so, and above the catcalls and roars of laughter I could hear, "Ride him, Doc, ride him," which did not add to my shaky confidence in the least. Fortunately I had brought a big heavy knife, or I never could have cut through that skin, which was like sole leather. Still more fortunately the poor mule did not seem to feel any pain. At any rate, all he did was to twitch his skin a little more. I could hear Abe, holding his head, talking to him, and saying, "Steady, old boy, go easy," and the mule would roll an eye at him and seem to understand. The crowd kept calling,

"Give him a drink, Doc," "Tell him about his father, Abe." Then I cut an artery that spurted blood up into my eyes, but I tied it up at last and, covered with gore, cut out the tumor and threw it down by my foot on the ground.

The sewing up was hard work, and at last, as I was tying the last stitch, a dog crept up and seized the tumor at my feet, another dog made a rush for it, and then there was a dogfight all over the mule. In the midst of the disorder, Abe made a slam at a dog, missed the dog, landed on my head, and off the mule I rolled in the middle of this welter of blood, tumor, and fighting dogs. This was too much for the crowd, and in a moment they were jumping down from the log walls of the corral and running to the center where they pressed close around the mule, tumbling over his body and making a horrible row. In the midst of this confusion, the dogs were kicked loose, and I was dragged to my feet dripping with mud and blood. A friend, with the best intentions, seized the sponge used on the mule and roughly passed it over my face, not improving my comfort and appearance. I had a glance at the faces around me. All wore a broad grin. The crowd went wild with delight and evidently had a splendid time, as I heard one old-timer remark, as he wiped the tears of laughter from his eyes, "Why hell! I ain't had so much fun since I trampled a skunk."

Two weeks afterward I heard the heavy rumble of an ore wagon as it passed my door, and there were Abe's four mules, their heads up, and with the slow ponderous step so full of power, they proudly strode along, their bells ringing, the red pompons bobbing on their heads, and my mule in the lead team as well as ever. Abe saw me and with a grin pointed to my late patient, while his little daughter beside him, her blond hair tossing in the wind, shouted and clapped her hands.

Chapter 15
A Cutting Affair

 I had, that summer, an experience of rather an unusual kind, since it had nothing to do with firearms; in fact, it might easily have happened in a city. It may have been different among the cowboys of Arizona and New Mexico, but at the time of which I am writing there was among the Colorado cattlemen a sort of code concerning any knife play. The cowboy of Colorado would shoot it out with revolver or rifle, but for some reason the knife was not considered the thing among the range riders and was rarely, if ever, used. In this case, too, a woman was involved, and as women held a high place in our regard—partly because there were so few of them—it aroused much excitement and culminated in a near lynching. In the light of my present knowledge, I believe the man responsible for the attempted murder was really insane, but in that time and place the various degrees of insanity were not understood. Hairsplitting of that nature was left for the future, and cutting a woman was held about as bad as horse stealing and was to be punished in the same way.

 I was just back from one of my professional calls at a ranch near by. My horse was saddled, and I was sitting on my porch with my wife and baby for a little talk before I turned my horse into the corral. Some three months before, a Mrs. More and her mother had bought a small cabin near my home, about one hundred yards away over the prairie. They were quiet people who intended to open a restaurant. The daughter was a fine-looking woman who, it was said, had left her husband in Wyoming and run away to our little place, out of the way as it was, to escape him. I had spoken to these people only a few times and knew very little about them.

A Cutting Affair

As I sat on the porch I could see their cabin very clearly across the prairie, and suddenly my attention was attracted by a man running out of this cabin, a large, powerful-looking man, a stranger I had never seen before. He jumped on his horse in a terrible hurry and spurred him to a run as he disappeared down a side trail. The next moment Mrs. More's mother burst out of the cabin, screaming and waving her arms to me to come over. She seemed crazy, tearing around and yelling out. I could make out, "Come, Doctor, come." So I ran over to my horse, mounted, and loped him over to where this frantic woman was screaming. As I dismounted she cried, "He has killed my daughter!" And seizing me by the arm, she dragged me to the door of the cabin and pushed me inside. I never saw such a mess. The table, with dishes and food on it, was thrown over, and the broken dishes were scattered on the floor. This room was used as a kitchen and bedroom in one. The ceiling, made by stretching sheeting from the walls, was very low, just above our heads. In the struggle it had been torn down, and was hanging in long strips, dripping with bacon fat and blood, while the walls were splashed in the same way. On the bed, where the blankets were half pulled off onto the floor lay Mrs. More, all huddled up, her hair falling over the side, one bare arm over her head and cut to the bone in two places. As I turned her body over I saw that her throat was cut, and she was unconscious and very white from the shock and loss of blood. Pushing her mother aside, I got my surgical kit from my saddle and, while her mother held her head, I tied off some of the bleeding blood vessels and put in a line of stitches to close the wound in the throat. I was glad that the cut was not deep enough to injure any big blood vessel or really endanger life. While I was bandaging her neck and arm she recovered enough to smile at her mother, and in half an hour she was sleeping.

I then took the opportunity to ask the mother for some more details about the affair. We went outside that we might not disturb the patient, and I was told by the mother that her daughter had married this man More some years before, and there was born one son, now with relatives in the East. More was one-eighth Osage Indian, a very powerful man, of violent temper, and he had led her a terrible life with his jealousy and fits of rage. He had been working at a ranch in Wyoming. Six months before, she had run away from him, joined her mother, and had come to our little place, far away from everything, where they hoped to be safe from this violent man's revenge. They had heard nothing about More since she had left him, and then, to their terror, he suddenly appeared, jumped from his horse, and entered the cabin. He was excited and evidently bent on any kind of violence. The poor women, who were alone and helpless, watched him in silent terror, as with vile curses and threats he asked his wife if she would come back to him. The mother replied, "No, I would rather see her dead!" This seemed to make him furious. He rushed over to his wife, who screamed and backed up against the bed, half falling onto it, as he caught hold of her hair in one hand and slashed at her with a knife in the other. As she threw up her bare arm to protect her neck he slashed it across to the bone, then twisting her arm down, he

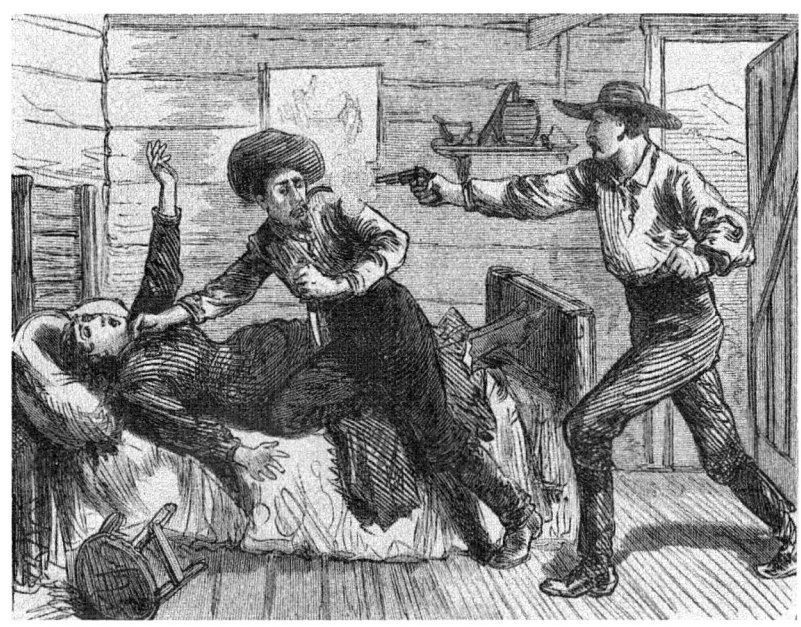

A Cutting Affair

cut her throat. At this, the mother, a frail little woman, who had stood paralyzed by fear, seeing her child being murdered, and hearing her cry out, "O Mother, Mother!" in desperation seized the only weapon at hand, the frying pan on the fire, and, with all her strength, brought this frying pan down on More's head again and again. He staggered back half blinded by the blow and hot grease, and, believing he had killed his wife, ran out of the door and galloped off on his horse. During the struggle the blood was splashed about, the pan had caught the cloth ceiling, ripping it down, and grease was splashed everywhere. The poor mother, when More galloped away, tried to help her daughter, who had fainted. Then, remembering how near my home was, she ran out and called me at the top of her voice.

I now wondered what to do, and decided to hunt up some men and round up this woman cutter. So I mounted my horse, and, seeing a few of the boys at the livery stable only about one hundred yards away, I rode over. The news had got out someway, while I was treating Mrs. More, and I saw men riding off and entering the timber down by the river to head the men off. As I reached a group of men by the livery stable they called out, "Look at the doctor." In my excitement I had forgotten that I was in an awful mess, with grease and blood all over my face. I got off and washed my face and hands in the horse trough, while I answered questions. Two of the boys ran down to More's cabin to guard the woman in case the husband came back.

And then Gus Wilson, foreman of the Lazy T outfit, rode up. Gus cried out, "A kid just saw our man headed for old Mead's ranch. Come on, Doc, we're the only ones with horses here."

Some of the men called, "Good luck, Doc," and held my horse when I mounted.

There was nothing to do but gallop after Gus, who was far down the road by this time, and I soon caught up with him and, as it was only three miles, we were at Mead's cabin in no time.

Mead, a man respected and liked by all of us, was an old bachelor, living all alone, a sort of retired cattleman. He was well off, and his cabin was substantially built and as neat as wax, while the yard was properly fenced. And there, by the cabin, was a horse all blown by hard riding. By a common impulse, we flung ourselves off our horses and ran to the door of the cabin where we heard voices inside, and then sounds of a struggle. We each had the same thought, that the murdering devil was about to kill poor old man Mead. Gus, with his rifle all ready, opened the door, and I followed him into the cabin. Upon looking over his shoulder, I could see two men on the floor, tumbling about and struggling so you could not tell one from the other. Gus caught hold of Mead and pulled him away, and the other man lay there, a hard-looking specimen that I knew at once was More, from his black hair and Indian features, with his head and face all covered with blood and grease. His throat was cut wide open into the windpipe, and the air, entering the wound as he gasped for breath, made a whistling sound. I saw that he was bleeding very badly, and when Gus got my instruments from my saddlebag, I knelt down on the floor and tied up a few blood vessels. I felt queer at seeing another throat wound so soon, but quickly found that he was not cut very deeply, mostly in front over the windpipe, while the big arteries and veins at the side had escaped injury, although it was a horrible wound. He was quite weak and could not talk until I closed the opening in the windpipe by a tight bandage around his neck, and then he whispered to me, "Is she dead?" Old man Mead was quite knocked out by the struggle and excitement, and had a bad cut in one hand. I dressed his hand and washed his face.

He said he was reading an old paper by the window when this wild man, whom he had never seen before, came galloping up to his gate, jumped off his horse, and burst into the cabin, his face all covered with blood and sweat, and no hat on his head. He had a knife in his hand and acted as if he was crazy. He yelled out, "Hide me or I'll kill you." It is not surprising that old man Mead, living all alone, was terrified, believing some crazy man had escaped and would kill him.

Without thinking, he rushed up and caught hold of the man's arm, trying to get his knife away from him. In the struggle they both fell over a rocking chair, and the first thing Mead knew, as they rolled on the floor, his face was covered with blood, and he thought the crazy man had cut him, but just then we came in, and he saw that the man had cut his own throat, and that he was cut only in the hand.

More lay on the floor, groaning from time to time. Then Gus said, "Listen," and down the trail to the cabin we heard horses coming at a run, and in another minute five of the boys pushed into the cabin, calling out, "Where is he?" They saw him and drew back a little, then one said, "Come on, boys, we'll hang him right now," but at this, old man Mead put up a regular howl, saying he would have no lynching on his place for it brought bad luck. Gus said he was running for county sheriff next fall and the boys would get him in bad if they did anything about lynching and he was one of the party. They were only halfhearted about hanging a man in More's condition anyway. All talked and argued together, and finally it was decided to take More back to town.

There was no road, so we had to take him on a horse. I tied up his neck as well as I could, for his head kept falling to one side or the other where the muscles were cut. We at last got him into the saddle. Sandy McGennis, a horse wrangler, got up behind him and held him up, with a puncher on each side to help. We could go only at a walk and made a strange procession. We were joined by other riders from time to time, and when at last we really got into town, all the people in the place, some one hundred or more, were waiting for us. Fatty Murphy, the blacksmith, in a red shirt, with his leather apron on, was out in front holding a rope, and yelled out, "Get him off that horse. We're going to hang that woman cutter now."

Things looked bad. I was awfully upset. I could not stand seeing this poor, half-dead wretch hung up, and yet, the temper of the people was so aroused I hesitated to interfere. But Gus was afraid of nothing and equal to any emergency. Pushing his horse in front of the prisoner, he gave a straight talk to the crowd, saying he was aiming to be sheriff, and that right now he was going to stand for law and order.

This gave me courage. I was so scared I could hardly talk, but like most timid people, I felt ashamed of being afraid, and so pushed my horse alongside of Gus. I heard my voice, loud and clear, as if someone else were talking. I do not remember all that I said, but I gave it to them in good measure and ended by reaching over and taking off the bandage around More's throat. His head fell back, and he was a tough sight. Then I said. "You can't hang him. He can breathe through that hole in his windpipe below the rope!"

Some wit in the crowd broke the tension by calling out, "Let's turn him over to the doctor. That's worse than hanging."

A few laughed, then all laughed, and in a moment the curious psychology of the mob changed, and to my surprise they now assisted us. A few still grumbled and cast ugly looks at us, but that was all. So we took More off the horse and carried him to our little cabin jail, while the people calmed down and went away. The lynching never took place. Had his wife been killed, it would have been another matter; but I told them she was sure to recover, and then Gus's talk broke the ice. I only followed him, but I have always wished that I had not waited but had been first.

We had a guard over More day and night for nineteen days. I had to operate on him several times. The wound became infected, and he nearly died, but he was a splendid, healthy animal and took a lot of killing. The blacksmith, who was so eager to hang him at first, came over to the side of law and order, made handcuffs and leg irons, and More was chained to his cot all the time. More was angry at me and tried to hit me, even fastened as he was; so I had to have two men hold him down when I dressed his wounds. He was sullen all the time. Why he had it in for me I do not know, but kindness did not have any place in the savage, perverted character of this man.

When a sheriff came from the county court and said that the trial would take place there, sixty-five miles away, I was served with a court order to take my patient there and also to be a special witness at the trial. More was about well by this time and, though he still spoke in a husky voice, his general condition, in spite of his confinement, was such that he could stand the trip safely. So we piled up a lot of hay in a wagon bed, put More on the hay, and tied his irons to the wagon bed. To tell the truth, we were all afraid of him. In the first place, he weighed two hundred and fifteen pounds, was six feet two inches tall — a mass of lean muscle. Then he was part Indian, and a sullen, ugly brute, bursting into rages, tugging at his irons, and yelling curses at us. The guards with me were good, quiet punchers, law-respecting men, chosen because they were steady workers; but in that drive of three days there were times when these men just about reached the end of their patience, and I still believe they would have hanged him if I had not talked them out of it. It was a mean trip, raining, and the road rough and slippery, so it was a relief when at last we reached the county seat and turned this evil-minded person over to the jail officers. I took the trouble to inform the officers that the man was a dangerous character and would bear close watching, but the only thanks I got was that no doctor could teach them how to handle bad men. So it was with much secret satisfaction that I heard the next morning that More, in an unguarded moment, had smashed one of these smart gentleman-guards a blow on the nose with his handcuffs that nearly knocked his fool head off.

The court, as might be imagined, in those unsettled times was conducted with scant regard for ceremony. The proceedings were held in a bare hall, constructed so carelessly of fresh lumber that the cracks in the walls freely admitted light and air, giving good ventilation at any rate; the only drawback was that any gentleman not wishing to be observed in court, had merely to squint through these cracks from the outside, and from this safe position would frequently interrupt the proceedings of the court by profane and personal remarks regarding the judge or jury, which irregular behavior drove the sheriff nearly to distraction.

The interior of this hall of justice was simply, if not luxuriously, furnished with benches, two tables, four or five sandboxes for the tobacco chewers, and a pitcher of water with a glass for the judge. When I arrived to be sworn in I had a few moments to wait, and was amused at the free and easy air. The judge, with the long-faded Prince Albert and big hat, looked the part of a frontier judge to perfection, and when with a "How are you, boys," he settled himself to work by thumping his big boots on the table, spat with much skill into a sandbox ten feet from him, and tilted his chair back at a comfortable angle, it all looked so like a play I had seen of frontier days that I could scarcely realize that it was reality. I noticed with some misgiving that More, the prisoner, was unshackled and attended by only two guards who sat one on each side of him. I was called up before the court, sworn in, and instructed to give my testimony. More's lawyer made much of the fact that More said he remembered nothing at all about the attack on his wife. It was all a blank in his mind. I testified that More had asked me, when I was dressing his wound, "Is she dead?"—meaning his wife.

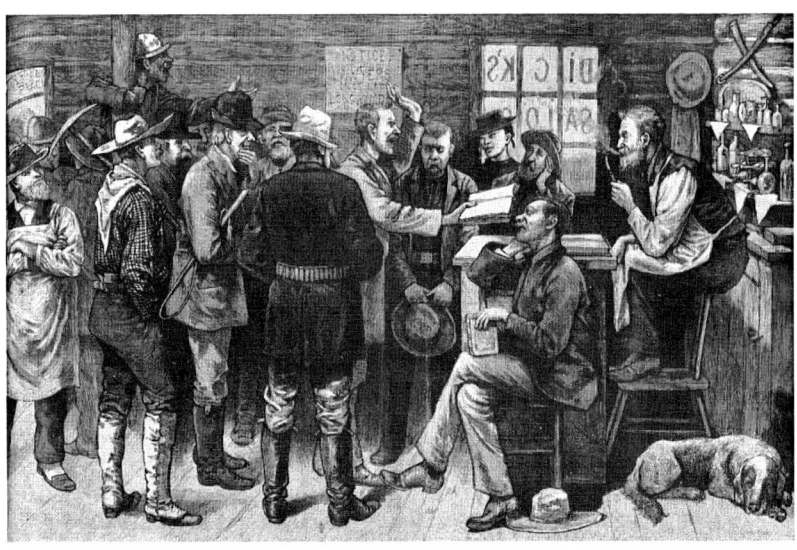

I did not think of the effect of this upon the prisoner. It clearly showed that he was lying, and did remember cutting his wife. My testimony made a stir, and I could hear the hum of voices and the cries of "Silence!" as I returned to my seat on a bench in the middle of the room about ten feet from More. I had barely taken my seat when More sprang up, calling out,

A Cutting Affair

"I will get you, you d—— doctor," and made for me, with the two guards hanging onto him, but such was his strength that he pulled these guards along with him as if they were boys. I saw More's lined faced cursing at me, his eyes like those of an animal, wild with rage. I knew how powerful he was. I could not run back over the long benches to the rear, and I was badly scared. I pulled my Colt .45, aimed for his chest, now almost on me, and was pressing the trigger when More and the two guards stumbled over a box, falling on the floor so I could not shoot without hitting one of the guards.

Moreover, by this time, a dozen spectators had flung themselves on the struggling men, and More was tied up, for the moment harmless. I was so excited that I did not see all that happened around me in the courtroom, but there was at once a wild confusion. Many thought that a rescue of the prisoner was being made, others that a general fight was about to begin. Men shouted and ran for the door, several hid under the benches, and the dignified-looking old judge snapped his feet off the table, pulled his gun, and was ready for action with a speed of motion acquired only by long practice. Of the twelve jurymen, eleven were seen to pull their guns promptly, while the twelfth vainly

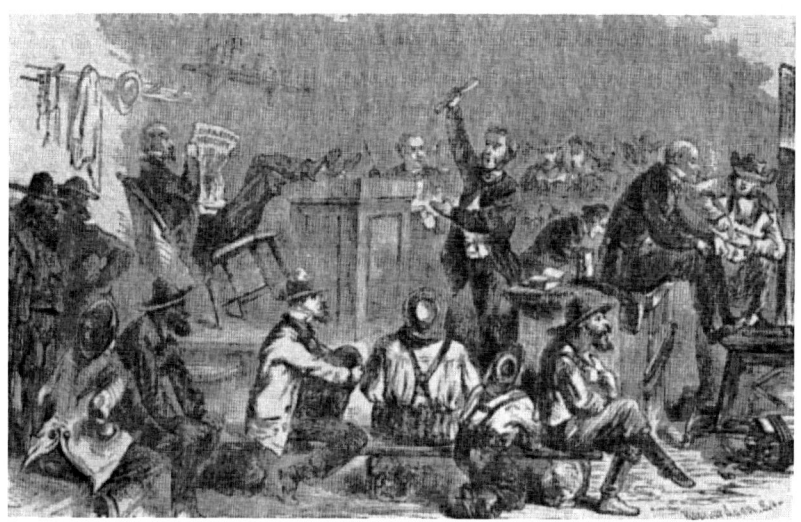

tugged to draw his, but it had caught on his suspenders. It was a lively time while it lasted; one never knew when a shot would start things, but at last the judge rapped for order, resumed his comfortable attitude, and the case proceeded. It went to the jury and they rendered a verdict of guilty and recommended fifteen years in prison.

I never saw More again, but as he was being taken out of court, closely guarded by a score of deputy sheriffs, he turned and again made threats to kill me.

The judge, addressing me so that the court could hear, said, "Doctor, we have all heard the threats this prisoner has made to kill you, and I wish now to state before this court that if at any time you may meet this prisoner, you have the sanction of this court to kill him at sight," which remarks seemed to meet the approval of several present, as they showed by saying, "That's right, Judge. The Doc sure has a killing due him." I am glad to say that the occasion never presented itself.

It was with much relief that, my duties as physician and witness being over, with More safe in jail, I could return home, but it seemed that I never could get rid of this More cutting business, and the story seemed to have an uncanny way of reappearing in the next few years. Some two or three years later I had left my rough life and was settled in a small city. I was in the lounge room of a hotel, in a dinner coat. Dinner being over, we had gathered around the fire, and we were telling stories. A very agreeable Englishman, a mining engineer who had been all over our country, was one of our party, and had made several visits to our mining camps in Colorado. When called on to give a few of his experiences, he rather bashfully said, "The most unusual sight I ever witnessed in the West was in a boom town a few years ago. I entered a court room where a man was being tried for an attempt to kill his wife by cutting her throat. The prisoner made a rush for the doctor who had treated him, and I give you my word that the doctor, the judge on the bench, and the jury all pulled revolvers. I never could have fancied such a thing. Imagine, in a court of law! My word, but I lost no time in running out of the door! No doubt you will think I am drawing

A Cutting Affair

a long bow, but I assure you I was quite sober, and the thing happened as I say."

I could not remain silent, and very quietly I said, "You are quite right. I was that doctor you speak of."

For a moment the Englishman glared at me with a red face, evidently in doubt and anger, for I daresay, dressed as I was, he failed to recognize the cowboy-looking doctor of the courtroom.

Finally he blurted out, "I say, you know, are you chaffing me?"

I replied by telling him a few facts about the trial that convinced him, and very handsomely he got up and shook my hand, saying, "My mistake. So sorry. It is quite all right."

That fall a couple of my friends joined me in a visit to my old home, far from railroads, on a hunting trip. We were all in a coach, some twenty miles from a cow town where we intended to spend the night, when down the road ahead of us and coming toward us at a furious gallop, rode a woman whom, as she approached, I recognized as my old patient, Mrs. More. I called to her to stop, and, as she drew her bronco up, I got down and approached her. She knew me at once and breathlessly called out, "Oh, Doctor, More has escaped! I was warned today, and I am going to hide out. He will kill me if he finds me, and you too, Doctor!"

I detained her long enough to have her lift the velvet ribbon around her throat and allow me to examine the old scar, and then, with a "You made a good job, Doctor. So long," she was away at full gallop. My companions made some tactless remarks about beautiful women and cowboy doctors, and apparently derived much amusement from the neck examination I made, but I did not enlighten them.

I thought I was through with this episode in my life and had about forgotten it when, on a little holiday, as I was watering my horse at a mountain resort far up in the hills, a boy of about seventeen came up to the trough and watered his horse. The boy looked at me very curiously. He had black hair and pronounced Indian features. A big strong boy, he was. At last he said, "Say, are you the doctor —— who used to live in —— ?"

"Yes," I said.

"Well," this boy continued, "Mother has told me all about you—how you saved her life. I am Mrs. More's son. She raised me to kill that d—— father of mine, and I sure am a-going to. He's in Creed, and I am on my way." Before I could question him further he was off.

I never heard anything more of this devoted family, and fortunately I never ran across More again.

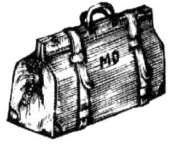

Chapter 16
"Ranch Jumping"

After the trial I found the county seat much excited over a boom, caused by the grading for a railroad that was now sure to come in a few months. All kinds of people were crowding the town: miners, cowboys, land sharks, and the large force of men on the grading job. To me, fresh from the silence of the big range country, the crowd, as it surged from one saloon to another, the lights going all night, the dance halls and gambling joints wide open, the music of a German band making night hideous, and the general air of reckless adventure common to all boom towns, was an amusing sight.

This boom affected many people and in many ways. Saloonkeepers and gamblers, of course, reaped a good harvest while it lasted. Town lots jumped to hitherto unheard-of prices, for the first railroad into town would put the place on the map, and the grading for the right of way was being rushed through by hundreds of workers, only some twenty miles remaining to be completed. All this activity led to the wildest speculation, not confined to the town but extending all around it, even to the isolated ranches which, before this, had not been considered worth buying but now were eagerly sought. Titles to such lands were the cause of much trouble; disputes arising in regard to ownership often led to violence. Near the town were ranches with good natural hay lands along the streams, many of them belonging to old settlers who had failed to comply with the law.

As I remember, the law provided that, in case of land open to settlement, a man wishing to acquire a ranch, drove in a stake with his name on it, then went to the nearest land office and recorded his claim, had the land surveyed, and recorded that. The Government then issued his permit; the man was required to build a cabin and make certain improvements, such as fencing, and actually make the land his home for five years. At the end of this period he could "prove up," pay the Government $1.25 an acre, and get a regular title deed to the property. Many complied, but there were others who were careless, and among these were some of the very first settlers, who had gone into the country, made a camp where they had found some stream, with grass, timber, and water; later, a cabin was built, a living was made by hunting and trapping, a few horses and cows were collected, pasture was fenced and, in short, a ranch was developed. Never having taken the trouble to have the land surveyed or entered, they felt that, as they had been first on the ground, the land was theirs, and, law or no law, they would hold it against all comers.

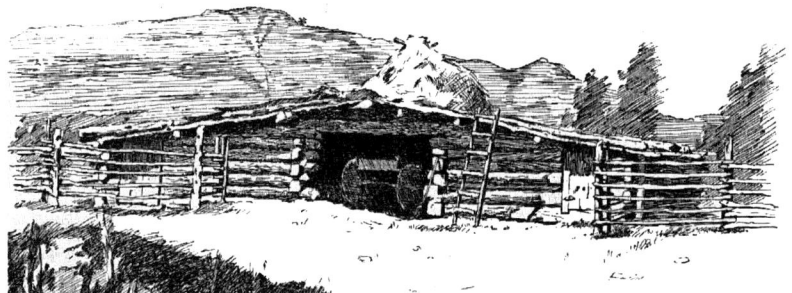

There was a certain amount of sympathy with these lawless settlers among the few ranchmen scattered here and there over the region, and no one disturbed them; after all, they had really been the first to open up the country. It was held as an unwritten law that these places did belong to them by right of discovery, but with the coming of the land boom it was a different thing. Crafty lawyers got to work and found that some of the most valuable ranches were occupied by men who had no legal right to them, since they had not complied with the law of entry; therefore, their ranches were still part of the public domain, open to settlement by anyone who would drive his stake on them and record it at a land office in regular form. Many of these ranchmen, seeing "the handwriting on the wall," hurried to the land office and entered their land in the regular way, but others neglected to do this. It is

Ranch Jumping

easy to see what happened when some agent for a land company, arriving at the ranch of some fierce old-timer who had fought Indians to hold it, told the ranchman that the title to the land was not his, as he had supposed, but was vested in the agent.

To make things worse the law was utilized by a political ring in Denver that used any means to obtain land. It was during this time that the powerful political party in Denver conceived the brilliant idea of recruiting certain lawless and wild Irishmen — who had probably found Ireland too hot to hold them — as agents to further their schemes, by paying them to "jump" ranches that were settled by men unable to show a clear title. The Irishmen, out of work and desperate, were willing to take big chances, for they were well paid for this work. Often, when they asked to be protected, they were aided by a deputy sheriff, and, as the power of the politicians extended far and wide, even local officers of the law were under their orders, but some sheriffs were of the old stamp and refused to help anyone against their old friends.

It was in a shooting affair caused by these unsettled conditions that I came very unexpectedly to play a part, and take on duties not ordinarily a part of a physician's work. At that time and place a doctor was frequently forced to face some amusing situations — and some not so amusing.

Called out of court where I was a witness in another peculiar tangle in which my professional work had involved me, I was greatly surprised to be told by a number of excited citizens that there had been a shooting up Clear Creek and a doctor was wanted at once, for three men had been shot. The local doctors could not be sent. Of the three doctors in town, two had gone out to an accident at a grading camp, and the other bright light of the medical profession was so drunk he could not stand up. So I got excused by the judge and rented a pair of horses and a light buggy from the livery stable. My broncos were not shod and had tender feet from the seventy-mile trip the day before. As I climbed into the buggy, the liveryman said, "Can you drive some, Doc?"

"Yes," I said, "why?"

"Well," that worthy replied, "that team you got is a good team, but it ain't broke gentle yet."

This encouraging remark made me a bit careful in driving, but all went well until I came to a place where the road was cut out of the bank above the creek for several miles—a sheer bank on one side and a drop into the creek on the other side. Like all new roads, it was rough and narrow in places, and there were turnouts where, by crowding, you could just pass if you met another team. It was, of course, at this precarious stretch of road that a big jack rabbit suddenly darted under the feet of my horses and, with a bound up the steep bank to one side, kicked dirt and stones into their faces. Both horses reared and cramped the wagon around so that one rear wheel hung over the bank above the creek. I did the only thing possible—cut the team with the whip—and they at once ran away; down this narrow road they tore, rounding corners, the hind wheels throwing stones into the creek, grazing the bank by inches; and all my pulling on the lines of no use except to make things worse, for the horses kicked back when the buggy crowded up against them. Once I caught a blurred picture of a wagonful of people drawn into a passing place, all the people with open mouths as I flashed past. A dozen times I just missed plunging into the creek fifty feet below; then the team, exhausted, finally reached more open country, and I got control again.

This was a trying experience, and I was glad when at last I saw a small log cabin down by the creek. Men were crowding around it, and riders heavily armed were riding up and dashing off again, so I felt this must be the place where my wounded men were. I was greeted by the Irish settlers with much good will, my team unharnessed and put in a shed, while I entered the cabin to find it crowded with an excited mob, all carrying rifles, all talking at once, while confusion, fear, and anger were written on all the faces. These Irish settlers, in their rage, were shouting violent and terrible threats against the man who had shot and wounded the injured men. They were searching every trail for him, and were so excited that I could get no connected story of what had occurred, only the cry, "We'll lynch the murdering devil."

When I had driven most of the men out that I might make a proper examination of these patients in some peace and quiet, I

Ranch Jumping

found a man sitting on the only chair while friends were putting wet cloths on his ankle, which was black and swollen where a rifle bullet had hit him a hard smack, but had not entered. In one end of the cabin was a regular old four-poster bed, big enough for four people, and evidently an old family heirloom. Upon this bed lay two men, young fellows, groaning with pain and calling on the saints. One was hit in the chest, the bullet breaking his right collarbone and then ranging down to come out at his back. He was having hemorrhages from his lung, the pieces of collarbone having been dashed into the lung by the force of the bullet. The other man had been on the reaper when hit, the bullet cutting across his abdomen and his intestines coming out; and yet, with this fearful wound, he held his intestines with one hand and drove one hundred yards before he fell fainting from his seat.

I saw there was no hope for these poor boys, and called some of the older men and told them. They knew it anyway, but told me to go ahead and do all I could. Their only complaint was that there was no priest who could arrive in time. I sewed up Pat, who was shot in the abdomen and, fortunately, he felt very little pain; he was almost unconscious from shock; but Tom, who was shot in the lung, was growing very weak. He told me his mother's address in Ireland, and I promised to write to her. I took down his ante-mortem statement, for I knew I should be called upon to testify later. The poor boy knew he was going, and thanked me before he died, some two hours later. The other man, Pat, was unconscious and died at nine o'clock.

The men stayed with me until then, but a man riding in said that they had located the man who shot the boys, and wanted all the men to come and surround the place; so they all saddled and rushed off, leaving me alone. They said another party of settlers was coming in soon, so I should be alone only for a short time; but by some mistake no one did come, and I was alone all night, for the man who was hit in the ankle was driven to town in my buggy, and I was glad to see this runaway team out of sight.

I found some food and cooked a small supper for myself, and then I thought it was a kind idea to fix the boys up a little, for they were Catholics, and I knew they would have wanted to look decent. I found a razor and shaved them. I put a long board on each side of the bed so they would not sag down so much, and then covered each one with a blanket to keep the swarms of flies off. Then I lit two candles and put one on the board at each head.

The cabin was a small one and very old; the chinking between the logs was loose, and the ceiling was black and dirty with smoke and cobwebs. It was the cabin originally built on the ranch by Howe, the owner, who later had built and occupied a new cabin, a quarter of a mile away. When the Irish crowd took over the ranch by "jumping" it, they moved into the old cabin, although it was about ready to fall down on their heads, and when the creek was in flood it was always under water. Being in a hurry to cut the hay, they had made no repairs but were living there when the shooting occurred.

I cleaned up the place as well as I could, just to do something to pass the time. At midnight I could hear thunder and, before long, a thunderstorm blew up, flash after flash of lightning, with a regular cloudburst. The candles were blown out, and the rain came beating into the cabin between the logs. The cabin was on low ground, and soon the water poured through the doorway, and I was standing in water and mud. I sat on the one chair, but the legs sank into the mud floor, so I just slouched around in the mud, hoping the old dirt roof, weighing many tons, would not get so heavy that it would fall in on me.

Then the storm passed, and I lit the candles again. I wanted to write up my notes, but the one chair was of no use, for it sank in the mud, so I climbed over the foot of the bed and sat up against the headboard. There was plenty of room in the middle of the big bed between the bodies, and I had the light of the candles at their heads. It was the only comfortable place I could find to write. It was very uncanny and lonesome, and many have asked me if I were not overcome by horror at being all alone with the dead bodies. I did not feel very unhappy over this, for I was a doctor, and my training in the deadhouse at the hospital had cured me of any nervousness about dead bodies;

besides, the poor boys had thanked me. My conscience was clear, so that the impression in my mind was more as if they were friends. The flies, driven indoors by the storm, kept up a constant buzzing, and were constantly falling into the candles in a most annoying manner. They swarmed over everything, so that I could hardly write.

The dripping from the roof splashed on the bed, and the creek ran bankful, with a sound roaring above all else. The dark corners of the cabin seemed alive as the big log walls turned and twisted in the feeble and flickering light of the candles. The wind blew through the tops of the pines around the house; and they swayed and gave forth squeaks and groans up in the dark night overhead. At times a sudden puff of wind rushing through the spaces between the old log walls would, for a moment, seem to lift the silent forms on each side of me, and give them a startling and grotesque effect of coming to life, as the blankets rose in waves that rolled along from feet to head, a horrid and fearful imitation of a body struggling to sit up and then falling back as if too weak. However, I kept on writing in my notebook, putting down the main facts of the shooting.

Mr. Howe, a man of considerable education, and the superintendent of the first school, had settled in this little valley many years before, had built the cabin I was then in, fenced his meadowland, and raised cattle. In that year he had built a new cabin on his land up the creek. He had been called to Denver by the death of his father, but hearing of the land jumping, had hurried back only to find this Irish outfit settled on his land, cutting his hay. He had never recorded his claim. He saw lawyers and was told he could do nothing. The rough bunch of Irish was in possession and was upheld by the law. He felt outraged and insulted. The land that he had discovered, cleared, and slaved over was all that he had, except a few cows, and the hay from the meadowland gave him his income. To a man born and reared on the frontier, the unwritten law of the frontier was certainly in his favor. The crowd of emigrants had only just landed, and for them to come in and take all he had was a hard blow after he had made every peaceful effort to avoid trouble.

At last he decided to use force, if driven to it. Howe was no novice, for he had fought Indians and cattle thieves, had shot a rifle when he was too small to hold it and had to rest it on a log, and in spite of his quiet voice and simple modest manner, he was a bad man to trifle with. This fated morning he left his cabin and walked down to his meadowland, where he found three Irishmen, one driving the reaper and cutting his hay, while the others stacked it. All three were armed with revolvers. He told these men that the land was his, and ordered them off or there would be trouble. The men stopped work, laughed, tapped their guns at their sides, and told him if he wanted to fight they would give him all he wanted; but they were now on the ranch. It was their ranch by law, and he must get out. Howe never said a word; he just walked two hundred seventy-eight paces to a corner in the field where two fences met (I paced this off later and testified to it at the trial), climbed a fence, and, turning around, rested his rifle on the top of the fence, took careful aim and shot the three men, one after another, and then took to the timber and vanished. One Irishman emptied his revolver at Howe, but missed him.

This was the story I put down that night. I grew sleepy in spite of the loneliness, flies, and the dead men. I was very tired but I tried hard to keep awake. The candles were so low I put them out and then slumped down in that gruesome bed and, before I knew it, was fast asleep. I woke with a start. The door stood open; the sunlight came in, flooding the darkness in turn. I was dazed for a moment, and then a big man walked in to the foot of the bed, and I saw it was the county sheriff, a big dark man in hip boots, armed like a battleship, a gun on each hip and a Winchester rifle in his hands. As he was, he looked a hard and dangerous man, for he was tall and large, his dark eyes staring sternly at me as I crouched, half-awake, between my rigid bedfellows.

"By gosh, Doc," he said in his deep voice, "I would not sleep in your place for a million dollars, no, sir!" As I crawled over the footboard to reach the floor, he pulled the blanket half off one of the bodies, and there, on the blood soaked shirt, I saw hundreds of big white maggots heaving and crawling over one another; the blowflies had been busy while I slept. As he tossed the blanket back with an oath of disgust, I brushed my clothes in a frenzy, and rushed out into the open air; I could feel those white worms all over me. I stamped and shook my coat to get rid of any chance maggots about me. Mr. King, the sheriff, followed me out, and, as we stood by his horse, he hurriedly said, "Doc, this all is a bad business. Howe shot these men, and the Irish are man hunting him all up and down the creek. Now I ain't going to have him lynched, and I just heard he's back at his cabin, a mile up from here, and you're the only man I can get to help me, so I call on you, Doc, in the name of the law, to come along and arrest Howe."

I was tired out; I had no breakfast; and the idea of taking that man by force, when I had seen the awful, deadly skill of his rifle fire of the day before, threw me into a cold sweat. I racked my brain for an excuse to back out, and then, in imagination, I saw the smile of scorn on the faces of some of my good friends as, standing up at the bar having their drinks, the story would be told of how "the Doc showed up yellow when asked to help King arrest Howe." I did not like the scene I saw in my mind's eye a little bit. I ran into the cabin, got my hat, buckled my gun on, saddled a horse in the shed, and was riding with King before I had time to think.

At last we saw Howe's cabin and came to a pole gate in his fence. I dismounted and lifted the poles down so we could go through. My old fears came back upon seeing a window in the cabin facing us, through which I expected a rifleshot to come every second. I could feel the bullet tear through me, as it had through the poor boys down in the cabin I had left. My legs shook so much that I could hardly mount my horse, and King, quite unnerved, remarked in a queer way, "Say, Doc, if I was as scared as you are, damned if I wouldn't run back."

Of course, that made me mad, and I was rude in my answer to him, which seemed to amuse him. We tied our horses and walked quietly to the cabin. More accurately, we crept along, half bent over, and took advantage of every bit of cover to keep out of rifleshot, and it was a relief when at last we crouched up close against the cabin, where no rifleshot could reach. I wondered why King did not call out Howe, but he explained that Howe might think it was a trick of the Irish gang hunting him, and go to shooting at once before King could explain who he was. King then said, "You guard the front door, Doc. I am going to the back door."

I rested my gun against one of the posts of the porch to keep my hand from shaking. It seemed an awful time. There was not a sound. Some birds sang as they flew about the bushes near my head. And then, with a crash, I heard the back door thrown open and the deep voice of King saying, "Howe, I arrest you in the name of the law!" and a quiet, gentle voice replying, "All right, Charlie, I won't make any trouble." My relief was wonderful. I felt as brave as a lion, and opened the front door as if man hunting were my joy and delight.

There at the table sat the outlaw I had pictured to myself as a killer, a small, very quiet man, with a gentle smile on his face, drinking coffee, and joking with King as if it were a pleasant morning for a call. As King introduced me, I found myself shaking hands with this desperate character as if it were all the most natural thing in the world; and more than that, as soon as he heard I had had no breakfast, in spite of my protests, he proceeded to cook flapjacks and make more coffee. In the most kindly way in the world, he forced me into a chair and waited on me with the most engaging hospitality and good manners. I felt as if I were dreaming. The talk was careless and humorous, and I soon saw that a stern sort of etiquette or code was being acted between these two men. No word was spoken of the shooting; it was evidently bad form to mention the subject; their relations were those of good friends; and yet, I realized that the sheriff would take this man to his death just as surely as the sun was shining, and that his prisoner, his word once given, would consider that word quite as binding as any chains or handcuffs, and any idea of escape would be a taint on his simple code of honor.

I made bold to ask Howe how he had dared to return to his cabin when he knew he was being hunted, and he told me in his pleasant way that he felt that it was the safest place to be, for he knew the men after him had been there several times to search the cabin, and would not think that he would dare return. Moreover, a good friend of his was leading the lynching crowd on a wild-goose chase that would leave him time to give himself to the sheriff. He also informed us that for some time he had watched us approach and would have gone out to meet us, but he was uncertain lest some of his hunters were in hiding and watching his cabin for a shot, so he calmly waited until King arrested him.

When King began to look restlessly through the window, and remarked to his prisoner that his Irish friends might think of searching his cabin again, Howe at once caught up his rifle, saddled his horse, and replied that he was ready. King seemed a bit embarrassed as he drew a piece of rope from his pocket and said, "I think, Howe, we had better make a bluff by tying you up in case some of the Irish see us." Howe mounted his horse, and King tied Howe's hands to the horn in front, all the time looking rather ashamed, then passed a rope around the neck of Howe's horse and, mounting, led Howe's horse after him. I noticed that the rope around Howe's wrists was very loose, only a slipknot, and also that Howe's deadly rifle was in a leather case under his leg, ready for action; so the whole prisoner business was a farce, to impress the would-be lynchers in case we met them on the road.

Howe seemed to appreciate this as he rode after King with a smile. King evidently intended the prisoner to help defend himself if an attack to lynch him occurred. Of course, I could see that King, although sheriff, was in sympathy with the prisoner. They were the same type, both old pioneers, and no doubt in his own mind the sheriff thought Howe had done only what anyone would do under the circumstances; but, being a sheriff, he knew duty came first, and he would bring his man in alive or dead, as part of his sworn duty, and no one knew this better than the prisoner, who, on his part, would never dream of attempting to escape once his word was given.

I was not feeling very happy over taking the prisoner to town, for I knew the Irish were out man hunting him for all they were worth, and what a small chance the law would have in holding back men as enraged as they were. My uneasiness was considerably increased when the sheriff said in his blunt way, "You ride back a piece, Doc, so if we rush them, you can hold 'em back." This was a nice prospect for a peace-loving medical man—to be shot in the back by a lynching party! However, I had to make the best of it, and our party certainly looked like a moving picture of the wild West as we rode up that valley. First came the sheriff, a big dark fellow armed to the teeth, his big hat just tilted enough to give him a regular bandit look of desperate courage. His boots came to his hips, and his big Mexican spurs tinkled like bells as he rode his nervous horse with that ease of seat and carriage in the saddle that is found only in men who have ridden from childhood. He led Howe's horse by a rope, and that prisoner, his hands tied to the horn of the saddle, rode by his side apparently as easily as if he always rode that way, while some distance back I came along in the doubtful honor of being the rear guard.

We all loped along at a good pace, for we were anxious to get out of reach of any lynching party. As we suddenly rounded a corner of the trail, we noticed three dismounted men standing there, all having rifles and evidently on guard to arrest our prisoner. My heart skipped a beat but, before I could realize anything, the sheriff gave a shout, and he and Howe just ran by those men like a streak. I saw one of the men raise his rifle as if to fire at the rapidly galloping figures, but his companions called to him to wait—and then I drew up right in the middle of them, the chills going down my back. I talked as fast as I could about the law's having its course, and said that Howe was being taken to jail, and so on, when one of the men said, "Why, ain't that the little doctor that laid out our boys so beautiful?" So all was well again, and there was no use in following the sheriff now.

Ranch Jumping

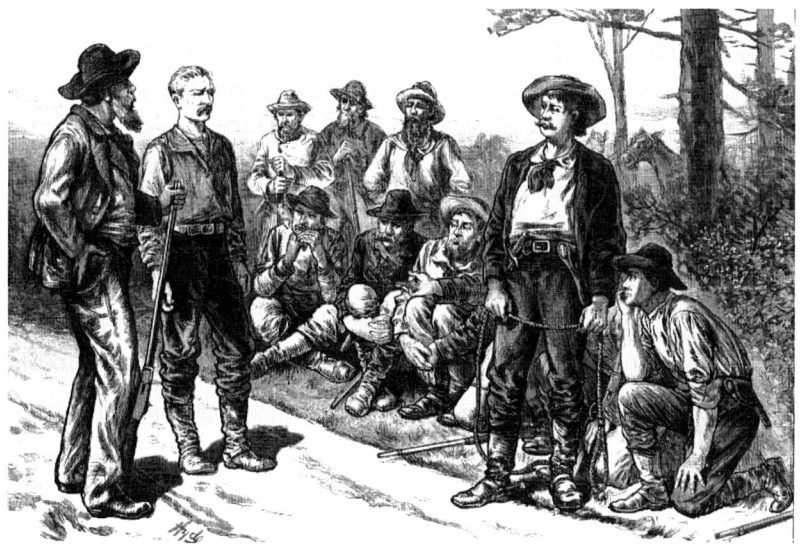

My horse was an old skate that could not get within a mile of them if I had tried to overtake them, and my new-found friends insisted upon my returning to the old cabin where the shooting had taken place. I was not anxious to see that miserable place again, but I felt that it was better to humor them, and I had to return my horse anyway, for I had only borrowed him. The cabin was all cleaned up, and the bodies in an outhouse, so I felt better when I got there, and I spent the afternoon with the others making two coffins for the poor chaps lying in the shed.

The next morning, in rode my friend the sheriff again, having delivered his prisoner in town. With him were the coroner and the jury that the inquest might be held at once. Such a jury—the outcasts of a boom town, loafers and gamblers, down-and-outers, two from the fair! As they crawled out stiffly from the two wagons that brought them from town, I thought I had never seen such a bunch of human wreckage before. King told me it was all he could get together, for good citizens were not to be found, and, as for making them come, when found, King inferred it was begging for a gun fight. The law, it appeared, did not function very smoothly at that time.

The proceedings at this inquest were marred, and much dignity was lost by the fact that no one knew anything at all about an inquest. The day was very hot, the long ride from town very trying to the thirsty gentlemen of the jury, and a jug of whisky in each wagon no doubt contributed to the general lassitude. The coroner and two jurymen had to be carried to the shed to view the bodies, for they were quite incapable of progressing in any other way. Then the "lit up" gentlemen, after very solemnly casting their bloodshot eyes upon the remains, at once entered into violent argument as to the number of dead they saw in the improvised morgue, two maintaining with much profanity that there were three bodies laid out. The third was equally positive that there were four bodies, all in a row, and ended his assertion by summoning the world to call him a liar.

When the sheriff had, with some violence, conducted these irate jurymen out of earshot, I proceeded to perform a post-mortem to show how the wounds produced death. Unfortunately, the weather was hot, the shed close and very

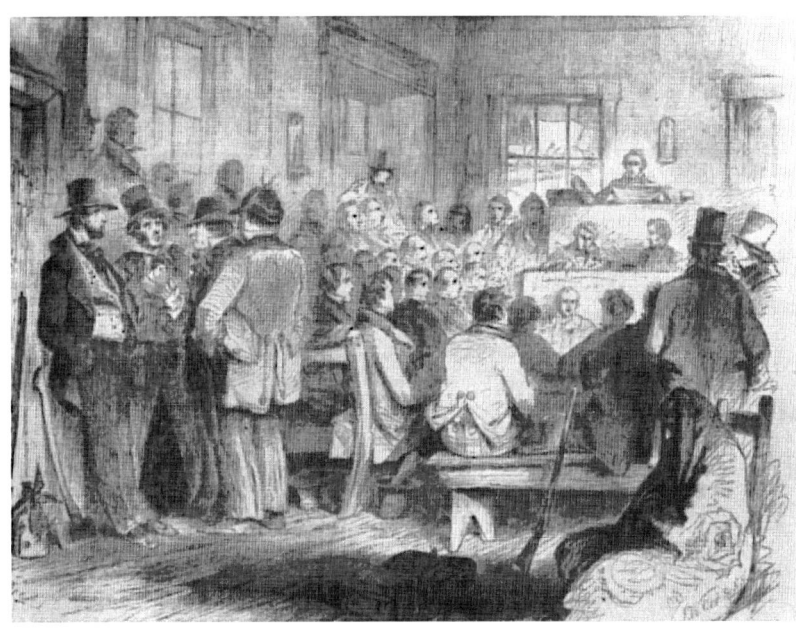

small, crowded as it was. The bodies had swollen, and when I opened one up, the gas escaped with a hiss like a locomotive letting off steam. The result on my spectators was immediate and disastrous to a degree. All, as one man, attempted to escape by the one small door, got jammed in the opening, struggled violently to and fro, and the frail shed rocked back and forth as if in a tornado. One of the bodies was pushed off the boards on which it rested and slid, passive and unresisting, into the lap of a gentleman sitting on the floor, very ill, who was engaged at the moment "pulling his lunch."

In fact, the inquest was not a legal success, and when I met the justly indignant sheriff, after the riot died down a bit, that worthy instrument of the law was in such a temper I feared to question him, for he was much engaged in loading the jurymen into the two wagons they came in and sending them back to town, unrepentant, and enlivening the way with ribald songs.

At last I got the bodies into the coffins and was told that the inquest would be held in town and, as a witness, I was asked to go along. So there I was, sitting on one of the coffins in a wagon, slowly rumbling our springless way along the road I had passed over so quickly in a buggy during the runaway. But now I was escorted by a cloud of flies that at times hid the horses from sight, and kept me busy batting at them with a branch of a tree all the long way to town.

At the trial, Howe was acquitted; I do not know the legal arguments used, but you could not find a jury at that time to convict him. The ranch jumping by the Irish settlers had a rude setback, and Howe proved up on his ranch in due form, and became one of the most esteemed citizens. I collected a little bill from the county and was glad to hitch up and pound the trail for home.

Chapter 17
"Jim"

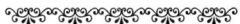

On one of my numerous hunting and fishing trips, I came across a little creek running into the river about sixteen miles below our small settlement and, prompted by curiosity, I followed this brook up three miles or more through the timber, having some trouble to get my horse over logs at times. At last I saw an opening in the trees ahead and suddenly arrived at a lake, some fifty yards across, made by the beavers. Their dam was still solid and held the water, but the beavers had gone long before. On one side of this lake there was a meadow covered with native grass and sprinkled with wild flowers, the paintbrush making a dash of scarlet amid the green grass. Around the lake the big white trunks of the quaking aspens stood in groups looking like canoe birch. Back of the lake the land rose in a mountain covered with pines, and down this mountain a brook ran among the trees and fell over a rocky ledge into the lake, making a small waterfall; and here, in the swirl of deep water, I could see native trout jumping out of the water as if eager to take a fly.

I fell in love with this little park and called it Beaver Park in memory of the cunning little animals that made the lake. Here was an ideal place to camp—good water for man and horse, wood all around for a fire, and fine feed for my horse. I could see no trace of man; the trails leading to the lake were made only by deer or elk; no trees had been cut by an ax; and the deer I saw were so tame, it was certain they had not been hunted. Here I camped and fished for several days. I shot only one deer. I never was a killer, and food for myself and dog was all I wanted. The beauty and silence of the place held me, and I selfishly kept it all to myself. That summer I made several trips all alone to my Beaver Park and brought home some big fish from the lake, all

Jim

wrapped in wet green leaves. They were so tame that I could use almost any fly, but it was grasshoppers, I remember, more than anything else, although a bit of red flannel was enough to cause a rush and splash, they were so eager. In late October it grew cold. I could imagine the park and the glory of the autumn as the leaves changed and were reflected in the lake. I had not been there since early summer and was waiting for a chance to go to my secret wilderness haven for some fall hunting when the deer are at their best and fat from mountain pasture.

Then, one day, a new settler drove into town, the family consisting of father, mother, and two children. As they drove up to our general store, the man got down and entered the store to buy supplies for the winter. He was a big blond fellow of about thirty-five, slow and lazy in motion and speech, a kind of "no good" I thought as I saw his shaggy horses and rickety wagon. I overheard him as he talked to the storekeeper, and told him he had taken up a bit of land by a beaver pond, was building a cabin and cutting a road through the timber to the river. My heart stood still. Could it be *my* Beaver Park he had settled in? Yes, there was absolutely no doubt about it; from his description I felt sure. I was half sick at the thought of this stranger breaking into this wild and lonely place, cutting down the timber, plowing up the meadow, catching all the fish, probably hunting the game away and, horrid thought, building a hogpen by the shore of my beloved lake! The grunting and smells in the pure and serene spot! It was too much, and I went out of the store mad and disgusted.

As I passed the wagon there was the wife, a frail bit of womanhood holding the reins, gaunt and yellow-faced — a worn-out drudge, too dull to care for anything; all work and no play, no woman to talk to for months, cooking, washing, childbearing, endless work, poor food — mostly pork and soggy bread. These poor sisters of the wilderness! They paid a price in winning the West, a price not noted by history, and only the very strong survived. Many were ailing and dragged along, hardly able to keep up. The pioneer doctor knew! The children were a contrast to their mother, dirty and in ragged clothes;

milk and the sun gave them their red cheeks and active bodies. When the little girl, as beautiful as an angel, smiled at me and, leaning over the side of the wagon with fun in her dancing blue eyes, called, "Hello, man!" I was won, in spite of the tragedy of my lost Beaver Park, and smiled back at the little woman as cheerfully as I could.

The family's name was Prime. Jack Prime came, some said, from Arkansas, and was a new settler in Colorado, as a small rancher. They drove away, back to Beaver Park, and I heard that the cabin was built, but paid little attention. In November a range rider belonging to an outfit on Piance Creek blew into my place late one afternoon and told me he had followed a wild steer belonging to his outfit clean up Beaver to the Prime place, and he found a sad state of affairs. The whole family were down with some kind of fever, the fire out, cold as blazes in the cabin, and Mrs. Prime calling out to him, "For God's sake, get a doctor." He did what he could, made up the fire, milked the cow, and then rode up to tell me. He was due at the home ranch and could not stop. I had to wait until morning, for it was dark as a pocket by this time, and I felt they were all right for the night.

At dawn I saddled up, put some food and medicine in my saddlebags, and loped down to the Prime place as fast as I could. The cabin was about one hundred feet back of the lake, made of cottonwood logs, half chinked with grass and mud, the dirt roof sagging already—a poor job all around. I pushed in the rickety door, and it was a sorry sight that met my eyes. There were two rough bunks filled with hay, father and mother in one, the children in the other. All were very ill with bad cases of typhoid fever. How they got it was a wonder, for

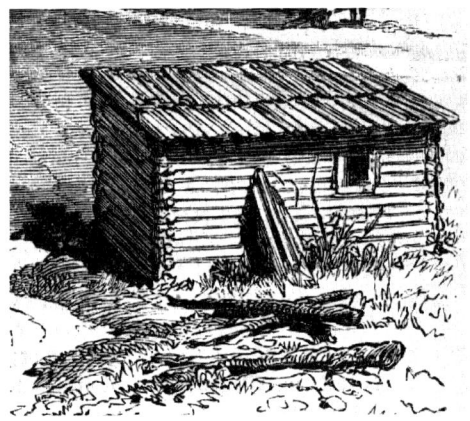

Jim

the water and food were all right. The poor people were in an awful state, just lying in filth, no fire, blankets soiled and half on the floor, the father muttering and half out of his head, with his wife trying to hold him on the bunk. Everything was tumbled about, the floor a mess with clothes, food, and dirty dishes. The poor children were crying and tossing about. I did all I could, got some milk, started a fire in the stove, gave medicine; in the afternoon I had to leave them, for I had a bad case at home.

I worried on that ride back, and in town at once tried to find someone to go down and nurse them, but had bad luck. All the men were away driving cattle down the river, and the few women left had small children they could not leave. One promised to go in a couple of days. I was up against it and started for Beaver Park again in the morning with my bedroll and some food so I could stay. My case in town was better, and I felt that I must stay by this Prime household for a few days anyway. As I passed the Prime corral on the way to the cabin I was surprised to see a strange bronco in the corral. A stock saddle hung on the top rail, and the horses and cows had been watered and fed. I thought some of the boys had heard the story and had come down before me. As I entered the cabin I found a strange cowboy cooking at the stove. He said "Howdy," and never looked up. I was astonished at what this man had done. The dirty blankets had been washed, new straw put in the bunks, and all the rubbish swept out, plates and towels clean, fire going, a pail of milk on the table, and the kids had clean faces; all done by this stranger, and never a word out of him!

Now there are two kinds of cowboys. Like other people they vary; some are jolly and full of talk, and others are the silent kind. This cowboy was the silent kind; I could see it written all over him. A tenderfoot would have said, "Well, it was kind of you to help these people. Where do you come from?" I knew better. By the code of those days he would have considered me just a chattering squaw and cursed me out or left me then and there. I did ask the woman, in a whisper, who he was but she said, "A stranger, just came in and started nursing us. One of the children asked him his name, and he said, 'Call me Jim';

but," she added, "that's not his name I am sure, and, oh, Doctor, he has been an angel to us!"

I looked at "the angel" and he certainly did not look the part. He had piercing steel eyes, a stern, lined face, a jaw like a bear trap, his mustache sunburnt a tawny yellow, tumbled hair falling over a face tanned like an Indian's, under the usual big puncher's hat, handkerchief around his neck, flannel shirt and blue overalls in his high-heeled boots. A small, wiry, bowlegged fellow, he moved about as if made of steel springs, in spite of a slight limp in his left leg. A man reared in hardship, he was a fine type of the old hard-boiled range rider, a lean, tough, outdoor man. I wondered, as I watched him, who 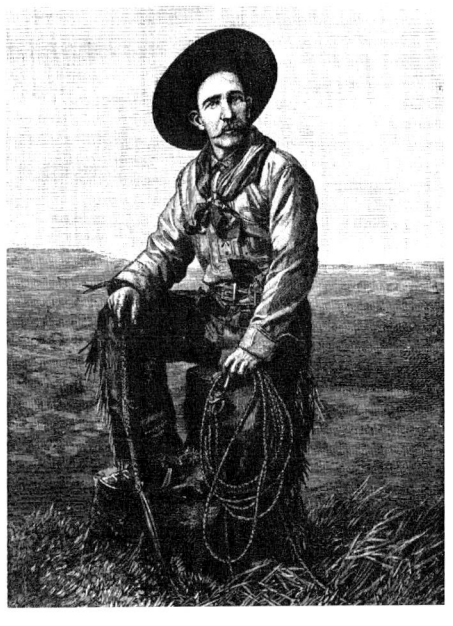 he was, how he got there, and why he was tending these sick people; but I kept still. I saw his rifle near the doorway and his revolver hung at his belt. He never took it off, and I just felt, "You are being hunted, young man; there is some history back of this," but it was his business.

As I left, we stopped a moment in the doorway. All he said was, "Get me some chewing tobacco, Doc," and then I saw his eyes harden and, as he quietly reached for his rifle inside the door I saw, on the other side of the lake, a buck and a doe. It was a good one hundred twenty-five yards, and the deer were now alarmed and flitting through the timber like silent phantoms. Now we could just see them as they passed by an opening between two trees, and then they were gone, to appear like a flash in another place; all this time they were bounding over undergrowth in long easy jumps. An impossible shot it seemed to me, but the next instant the crack of his rifle was close to my ear. The buck hunched up like a bucking bronco, ran for fifty yards, and crash! down he went. A quiet voice said, "I got him in the heart, Doc." I got my horse, and we went to the buck; there was the wound right through the heart, and I helped Jim cut up and pack the meat back to the cabin. I think he was pleased at my saying, "That's the best running shot I ever saw," but he never said a word, as was his way, and went on about his duty as he saw it, silent and faithful.

This mysterious stranger kept on caring for this family for five weeks, with never a word about his past or his reason for staying. I mentioned, in a casual way, that I thought some of the women in town could come and help now, but he flushed and was angry in an instant, so I let things ride as they were. This rough man was skillful in nursing, although probably never in his life before had he cared for a case of illness, unless it was of some horse, and when I showed some surprise at the way he shifted these bodies about on the rough straw to avoid their lying too long in one place and the pressure producing bed sores, he told me that a horse lying too long in one place got sores on his side, and he reasoned that human beings were much the same.

But what gave me the surprise of my life was to see how this simple puncher, bred among wild beasts and wilder men, never used to women and children, and far from all human sentiment as we know it, treated these helpless people. I fancied he would do his best under the difficult condition which he faced, and expected him to be kind in a crude, awkward manner, but, to my astonishment, I found this hardy puncher acting with an instinctive delicacy and tact that a trained nurse might envy. I was never tired of watching him as he tended these bedridden patients of mine. It was amusing to watch him, to see the different methods he used.

Men, in his mind, were one thing, and women another. As he took care of the father of the family he was abrupt, almost hard in his orders. It was, "Roll over, you!" or "Drink this"—no time wasted, orders were orders; and then, how his voice would change as he turned to the frail little woman! He seemed transformed into another man, his face softened, his hands grew gentle, and it was, "Yes, Ma'am. Just a minute, Ma'am." With what natural delicacy he covered her body, and with what tact he would try to make the embarrassing ordeal easier for her to bear, saying with his voice full of sympathy and respect, "Sorry Ma'am. Don't mind me, Ma'am. I ain't nobody, just a puncher passing through." And then, best of all, to see him with the children, no embarrassment when with these innocents, no need to act, just to be his natural self, so soft and gentle he was, handling these little wasted bodies. And when their fever grew less, and the dull stupor left their brains, with what skill he would tell them stories, always about animals, and always funny: what the mother fox did with her puppy, how a prairie dog lived in his home far underground. His whole face would change as a smile rippled over it, and the little thin faces, looking up into his, would change also. A light came into the dull eyes, a smile on the fever-parched lips, and for a moment the fever weakness faded away into the happier realms of health and sunshine. Of course, these children worshipped him, and my nose was quite "out of joint," my "nasty medicine" scorned at my hands, but in his rough ones, with a "Now, honey, be good," it was gulped down without a whimper. The mother, when she recovered, told me with tears in her eyes, of this strange man's devotion; as she lay awake in those long cold nights, suffering on the hard hay bunk, while the cowboy lay asleep rolled up in his blankets on the dirt floor, she would hear the fretful cry of a child calling, "Jim!" On the instant, up would spring Jim to give a drink, and a murmur of his low voice would reach her as he comforted the little one with stories, and then she could see his dim figure in the firelight as he sat by the bunk on his heels, as cowboys do, holding in that hard rough hand of his the soft and trustful one of the child, until restful sleep came again with Jim on guard.

This wiry man showed the strain of confinement and loss of sleep. His face grew thin, his frame gaunt, and I was worried over his condition. He had been for five weeks nursing and

Jim

caring for these people, and had very little sleep. The conditions in a cabin at that time are hard to realize now—no vessels for nursing, no rubber sheets. All the water had to be carried from the creek; a cookstove with wood provided the only heat, so that it was a constant struggle to keep clean and warm. With a disease like typhoid, the difficulty of nursing four patients, even in a perfectly equipped hospital, is very great; so one can imagine what this man had to contend with.

My patients were at last able to get about and help themselves, so I did not make a visit to Beaver Park for several days. Then, on riding down to visit them for the last time, I noticed that Jim's saddle was not hanging on the corral, and his horse was not there. I thought he had just gone for a ride, but, on opening the door of the cabin, the two children rushed to me and, clinging to my legs, cried out amid sobs and tears. "He's gone, he's gone," and I knew that Jim had left them. Each child held a beaded Indian belt tightly clasped in chubby fingers and with many tears told how they had found them on their beds when they woke up, the parting presents from Jim.

I think I know why he left like a thief in the night. The pain in those little hearts was more than he could stand, and he melted away into the wilderness, a coarse, violent man, but a very gallant gentleman.

The Primes moved away, as many pioneer drifters did in those days, to the El Dorado always just over the hills.

One summer I rode into Beaver again. The wilderness had claimed its own. The corral was broken down; the cabin roof had fallen in; growing creepers covered the windows, and on the doorstep lay a torn, crumpled rag doll. These fallen logs, once a home filled with childish voices, lay silent and deserted, and at dusk the coyotes struck their way amid the ruins, or howled in the moonlight.

Chapter 18
Some Hard Riding

On one of my long rides to see patients I had rather a curious experience, the tragic and comic being mingled in an odd way. This frequently happened in the old days among people far from law and order, living the primitive life amid savage and untamed nature.

It all came about from my friend Andy McKay's getting drunk, acting the fool, and, as a natural consequence, being rather badly shot up. Andy McKay was one of those curious persons you occasionally ran across on the frontier during that time, who defied any ordinary analysis as to character. Born in Scotland, evidently coming from a good family, he had received a sound education; but at sixteen he came to America to better his condition. The cities in the United States appalled this healthy Scotch lad, used to the open country and farm life of Scotland, so, like many another adventurous Scotchman, he soon left the restraints of civilization and came to Colorado. Of wonderful physique, tall, quick, and as strong as a horse, he soon became a cowboy. His knowledge of horses and his education gave him a decided advantage, so before long he was ranch foreman and had collected a little bunch of livestock he could call his own. He had, unfortunately, a quick temper which had involved him in some trouble, so that he hid out among the Ute Indians for a number of years. He gained a considerable knowledge of the language, married a couple of squaws, and was a "white Indian," respected and liked by the Indians. When I knew him he was in charge of the cattle at the Indian Agency. In this position he was not only very capable, but, because of his relations with the Indians, he was of actual service to the Government when trouble with the Indians threatened.

Some Hard Riding

Personally, Andy was a most likable fellow and, in spite of the stigma attached to the name "squaw man," was so square in his dealings with Indians and cowboys alike, that he had lived this down. He had accumulated some property in the shape of horses, and made his home among his Indian friends, living in a tepee with his wives and numerous half-breed children. With true hospitality he put me up on several occasions. At such times I was interested and amused to see how this educated Scotchman lorded it over his red brothers, and lived in a style probably closely resembling that of his ancestors, the Scottish chiefs.

His dress was a strange compound of Indian and white man—a cowboy hat, a shirt and trousers of soft, tanned buckskin, fringed and beaded, but with cowboy boots, and with belt and revolver like any puncher. He made a striking figure presiding over his home. His long blond hair falling to his shoulders, his erect carriage and look of command, made a most picturesque and unusual impression on the stranger seeing him for the first time, and, what with his large tepee, colored red, his big herd of ponies, and Indian relatives all got up with barbaric riot of color, it was quite a treat to enjoy his hospitality, especially since in the matter of food he still clung to white man's ways, dining on the best cuts of venison, sage hen, or mountain trout, not to speak of real old Scotch whisky.

It was months since I had seen Andy, for he lived some one hundred thirty miles south of me, near the Agency. There was a place down the river seventy-eight miles from my house where he came to trade horses. This place was in an arid region—

nothing but big rocks and canyons—and as hot as an oven in summer. Here a man called Tom took up a ranch. It was rather a joke—taking up a ranch in such a miserable place—but Tom's ranch, as it was called, raised "nothing but hell," as the boys said. It was near the river which here lost all its beauty and became a dirty, brown stream full of mud and alkali, in vivid contrast to the beauty of the clear water and the woodland parks on the banks above, through which it flowed. Tom, however, was not discouraged by the ugly prospect. He built a trading store, which was also a saloon and gambling joint, with a corral for horses, and a scow to ferry people to the other side of the river, for the trail to Utah was on that side.

Tom did a good business, but his place bore a bad reputation, many fights occurring in his saloon when men were shot; and some darkly hinted that Tom's place was simply a hangout for horse thieves, and that Tom himself was hand and glove with the outlaw bands that infested that part of Colorado. Anyway, this place was lawless enough, being over two hundred fifty miles from a railroad and frequented by men who were as wild and relentless as the wilderness around them.

At dawn one hot day in July, a rider for the Lazy S outfit galloped up to my place and told me that Andy had been all shot up in a gun fight down at Tom's ranch.

This rider had not been there but was told by a messenger who, his horse having given out some thirty miles below us, had urged this rider to come for me, for Andy was near death and calling for me. I did not like the prospect; the heat down the river was a terror over the alkali plains, but I had to go, so I filled my saddlebags, saddled my best horse, and lit out over the trail south.

A funny old fellow, called "Smoky," because he was so dirty, lived all alone in a cabin thirty miles down the trail. Smoky made a living by trapping and horse trading, and the rider who called me told me that Smoky said I could change horses at his place. It was easy going this thirty miles, with trees for shade most of the way, and I made good time, but when I reached Smoky's place his cabin was locked and there was no sign of Smoky. However, there was a bunch of broncos in the corral, and I had to catch one if I wanted a fresh horse. I was not much good at roping, but at last, more by luck than by skill, I managed to get my rope on one and drew him up to the snubbing post in the middle of the corral. He snorted and played up a bit, as they will, but to my relief proved gentle enough when the saddle was on him.

The next thirty miles over the desert was about as tough going as I ever remember. The alkali plains, white as snow, glittered in the sun; the heat waves made the trail heave up and down before me, and I was dizzy and faint. I rode into the river when I could and wet my head and splashed water over my bronco, who was as shaky on his legs as I was on mine, and at last I struck a summer camp at Yellow Creek. There were three boys there; and if you want to know what kindness is, just strike a camp of old-time cowboys when you are about half dead. They would not let me lift a hand, but gave me coffee, saddled a fresh horse, and one of the boys, called Sam, saddled his horse and insisted upon going with me, for, as he afterward expressed it, "The Doc came in looking like he'd died on the way down and didn't know it, so I just herded him along to Tom's." I never could have made it but for Sam. All I did was to follow him in a kind of dream, with my eyes closed, and my head whirling around with the heat. I heard afterward that it was 103° Fahrenheit at my place that day, and what it was on the trail down in the desert I do not know, but not far from 115° Fahrenheit, I feel sure.

At last the cabins and store at Tom's ranch came into view, and I was helped off, so weak I could hardly stand. Tom was there to meet me, and as I sat in the shade of the store to pull myself together a bit, he gave his version of the affair that had occurred. Tom was evidently more concerned over the loss of trade because of the shooting than over the condition of the patient I was to see. "This is surely hell! My store is a regular hospital. Who can drink his liquor with four such half-dead ones a-staring at him?" he exclaimed, with much bitterness. "Why two men can't shoot it out like gentlemen, without killing nearly half the population, gets me." But Tom was better than his talk, for I found he had been doing all he could and had given up his own bed to the sufferers.

I was surprised to find four patients after I entered the store. There were four cots, all in a row, each with a man on it, and looking strangely out of place among the trade goods on the shelves, the long bar and bottles at one end. In the first cot I found Andy propped up in bed, and when he saw me he was so worn with suffering that he cried out like a child and begged me to kill him or help him at once for he could not stand the pain another minute. All his nerve was gone. I was fortunately able to relieve him, but the case was very serious, for a .45 bullet had entered the abdomen, torn through the bladder, and come out behind (the details too technical to explain here). He was also shot through the thigh and the ankle. His squaws sat on the floor by him and, since I could speak a little Ute, they soon understood my directions and were very faithful in following them out.

The next patient was a man called Toby; he was shot through the buttocks, and so had to lie on his stomach; but Toby was a funny chap, anyway, and cracked jokes at his own expense all the time I was treating him.

A boy of nineteen, a wrangler, and a fine rider, had, in his hurry to get out of range, run full tilt into a barbwire fence near the store, cutting his face and nearly losing an eye. He also was the comic type, and bore all I did with a humorous bravery that nothing could subdue.

My fourth and last patient was a professional brother who had been kicked by a horse and was in no sense amused by the experience; apart from bruises he was really all right, although he complained bitterly.

I at last gathered the facts of this surprising and unusual gun battle which had put four men out of business.

Andy McKay came up the river with his squaws, ponies, and retinue, and camped about a quarter of a mile from the store, hoping to have a little fun gambling and drinking, as was his custom at times. Leaving his camp in charge of his squaws, he rode over to the store and, meeting some congenial friends, they all had a few drinks and were engaged in playing Mexican monte at a table in the store when, as luck would have it, a certain man called Long-suit Taylor strolled in to see the fun.

Now, Taylor was a gambler, not a bad sort at all, as such fellows were often "on the square," but he had had a row with Andy some months before, and now, seeing Andy half drunk, he tried to go out that he might not risk another row. Andy, half-seas over, jumped up and, following him to the door, told him he was a coward. Then things happened all at once. The men clinched, each holding the other's gun, and turning and twisting, they wrestled all over the store in a fierce struggle to shoot each other. Both were powerful men and each was able to hold his opponent's gun away from a vital spot, but as they swayed back and forth, both men fired their revolvers, the bullets going wild and entering the walls around them. This shooting made the store anything but a safe place to be, and the noncombatants naturally tried to save their skins by rapid action.

Two punchers jumped behind a barrel of sugar, and it was as well they did, for two shots hit the barrel. Two got jammed into the narrow doorway, and my cheerful friend Toby was trying to shove them through when he was hit. The youthful horse wrangler, being young and active, at the first shot darted out through the door ahead of the others, and in his hurry and terror didn't see a barbwire fence in his path, but ran straight into it, and his face, sliding along the top wire, was cut clear open to the bone, one eye being nearly gouged out.

The fourth patient was a doctor from Ohio who, in all innocence of Western ways, was having a hunt from his camp twenty miles east, when he was surprised and rudely disturbed by a party of cowboys who insisted upon his coming to see Andy at once. Unfortunately, this Eastern visitor, not wise in the ways of range riders, and without tact, informed them that he was out for a rest and that he did not intend to be bothered by a lot of drunken cowboys and their shooting scrapes. The boys, explaining that it was a question of life and death, were very patient with him, but insistent that he should go, whereupon he got angry and told them all to "go to the devil."

Johnny Budd told me the story afterwards. "You see, Doc," Budd explained, "we all knew he was a strange bird and did not savvy us none, but Andy was a-dying and so we just threw a rope over the doc and tied him on a horse which we led along back to Andy's. The two boys which he had hired as guides, set up a holler, but knew better than to make any gunplay. We was all sorry as hell that his saddle slipped and he got kicked and drug a little on Blue Hill, but it was accidental and not our doing, and if he'd come along like a gentleman in the first place, there'd been no trouble."

My medical brother unfortunately did not see the affair in that light and denounced the proceeding in bitter terms, announcing that he would have the law on them. I had to explain at some length that if he tried any law business on men like these cowboys, he stood a good chance of being shot, so I left him in a more reasonable mood. He was only knocked about a bit, and his men took him away in a few days.

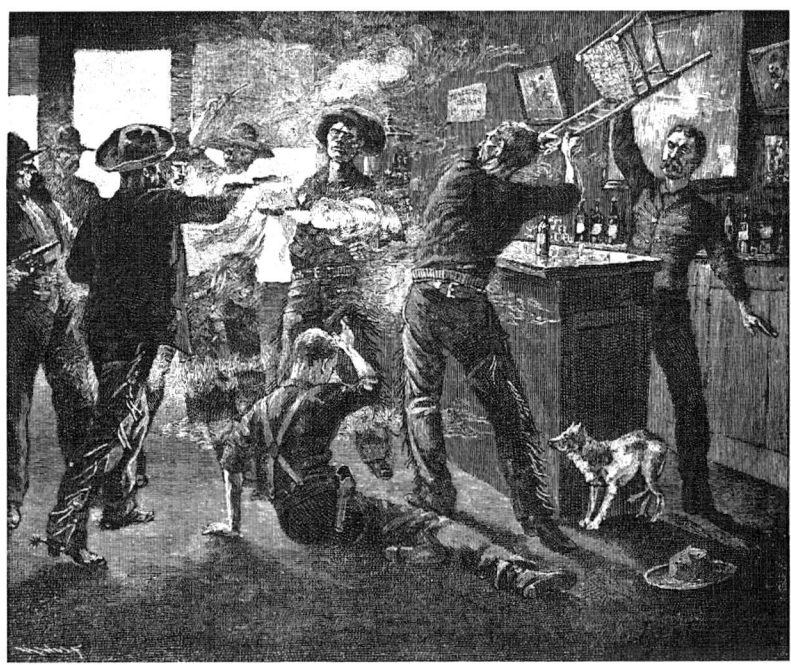

Some Hard Riding

I got the details of the gun fight from Andy later. In the struggle around the room, Taylor, by a sudden twist, got his gun free and fired low into Andy. Then Andy caught Taylor's gun again and pushed it down so that when Taylor fired again it hit Andy in the leg. Andy continued to push the gun down and the third shot hit Andy in the ankle. Andy was so weak now that Taylor jerked his gun clear and, putting the muzzle against Andy's chest, pulled the trigger, but his gun gave only a click on an empty shell, as he had fired all six shots. Taylor now ran through the door, mounted his horse, and rode away. Andy collapsed in a heap on the floor and lost consciousness. His squaws came running in from his camp and set up the regular death wail. The boys came back from hiding, and all hustled around and got cots for the wounded, sent riders out for the doctor who they knew was camped out east, while another messenger was sent for me. The affair created considerable amusement among cattlemen, especially the wound my friend Toby received in trying to get through the door. Toby was very fat and projected too far behind, but when joked about it, laughed with the boys and was voted a good sort anyway.

I had intended to stay at Tom's ranch a few days, for I was desperately in need of rest. I had to sleep on some blankets with no bed. The patients kept groaning and crying out all night, and my stomach was resenting the bad food, heat, and fatigue. At daylight a rider came loping up and knocked at the door to wake us all. He was in a mad hurry, and excited, for he informed us that a bunch of Utes had broken out from the agency and were coming up the valley raising all the hell they could, while a two-company post of United States Regulars had turned out some fifty miles below us. The officer in charge had ordered him to warn settlers all up the valley. With this pleasing information, he tore off north, riding as hard as he could go.

At this there was a regular stampede, men saddling up, and confusion everywhere. I was in a difficult position. I did not like to leave my patients, especially Andy, but I must go home to see about my wife and baby. I knew that there was a bunch of Utes hunting just above my home, and if Indian runners got to them and told them about the outbreak, they would not keep friendly long. I knew too that there were only a few men left in my home town, for most of them were in the hills after cattle, and it made me sick to think what would happen in a surprise attack by Indians. Andy was a rough man, but he just said, "Doc, don't you worry about me, I am safe and I can stand these Indians off from the others. I am related to most of them." And so this "bad man" told his squaws to bring his own horses, the best in his bunch, and when they put my saddle on one, Andy said, "Good luck," and I was away up the trail for home.

On the way back I was so anxious about my family that I had very little feeling about the heat and fatigue of the trip. I was possessed by the one idea of speed, and yet had sense enough left not to run my horses down and be left on foot. The first stage of twenty miles to my friends at a cow camp was taken at almost top speed on Andy's splendid horse. The boys quickly saddled a good tough bronco, and I loped along in a sort of dream until I reached old man Smoky's place. The old man was still away, but I found my own horse safe and sound, and when he nosed my pockets for sugar, it was almost like coming home again.

That last long thirty miles I rode in a horrible state of nerves. I did not know what had happened. I had met no one, and when I saw smoke ahead about where my house was, I pictured all the horrible tales I had heard of Indians. I suppose loss of sleep, and fatigue had broken my nerve. I soon saw that the smoke was from a forest fire on the oak ridge to the west, and when, about three miles from my house I met Albright, a rancher, who said that all was quiet at my place, I nearly fainted from the relief I felt. Albright laughed and said that the hunting Utes in our part of the country were all right, and had that day gone to town to trade, with their wives and children along; so my fears had made a coward of me, all to no purpose. I had just strength enough to unsaddle and turn my horse into the corral, to greet my little family, and fall onto a bed, dressed just as I was. I was too tired to eat, and fell asleep at once, and for the first time in my life slept for twenty-four hours.

Some Hard Riding

Andy McKay came riding into my place three weeks later. I often wish we could have moving pictures of those times to show people how the real thing looked. Andy was sitting sideways on his best pony, and one of his squaws was mounted back of him on the horse to hold him on. Then came several Indian friends and relatives, followed by his half-breed children driving pack ponies, with travois poles dragging behind, loaded with tepee tents, food, and blankets. Back of all, his pony herd was driven by Indian boys, with the usual collection of dogs and goats. They drew up and made camp near my place. The tepees with pictures on their sides, the bright colors of the Indian dress, their dark faces, with earrings and bracelets, beadwork, and feathers, all made a barbaric picture. Andy recovered in some wonderful way. I suppose I helped him with my surgery, but his wonderful constitution and Scotch ancestry, together with the devotion of his squaws, were, after all, the main things. He camped a week, for I still had to use some surgical methods on his wounds, and then they all went down the river again.

The last I heard of Andy was that he had settled in Old Mexico where, it was reported, he was running a big ranch for some New York men.

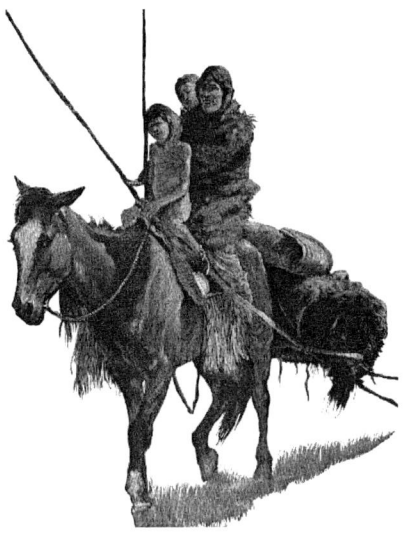

Chapter 19
Lawless Justice

All kinds of people came through our place; many were tenderfeet, not cattlemen at all, with no knowledge of the range, no skill, often with only a few cows. They built flimsy shacks to live in and hoped to sell out to the first comer. Not real settlers, they lived on the game they shot, went in debt, and were generally poor white trash. They did a lot of harm and some of them turned cattle thieves. They would round up a few calves, heat an iron, and put their own brand on them. This was easy and paid better than raising their own stock.

All this was small stuff, but it led to a serious condition. Real horse and cattle thieves from New Mexico and Arizona, as tough a bunch as ever lived, now began to operate on the larger ranches, driving off valuable horses and using such skill and boldness that we were up against it, for these outlaws were not only organized, but had spies that gave them all the news, telling them what ranch to raid next. The law was no help to us, for our country was run by a low bunch of political heelers, and it was rumored that sheriffs stood in with the outlaws, who paid a good price to be let alone. In fact, these outlaws, for some two years, ran the country so that a decent cattleman had no chance whatever against them, and the men who made any complaint were marked by the outlaws to be shot. I had a chance to see for myself what a lot of murderers these men were.

The Kelly brothers, good, hard-working boys, living all alone and doing their own work, had a ranch on a creek near our town, where they had some twenty head of horses. I often talked with the Kellys when they came to town to trade at our store. They told me they had done so well that they were soon going back East to marry their old sweethearts and make a real home on the ranch. Old "Shorty" rode in to our place one night, pretty drunk, with a pipe-dream story about the Kelly boys being blown up in their cabin. We all laughed at him, but in the morning he was sober and said he had the news straight. Squaw Charlie came along and, hearing the story, said, "Say, Doc, we ain't doing nothing. Let's ride down to the Kelly's and see for ourselves."

We rode down, and as we came in sight of the ranch down below us on the creek, Squaw Charlie grabbed my arm and said, "Look at the roof, Doc!" And sure enough the heavy roof of the cabin, made of logs and dirt, had been torn off. We rode up and, leaving our horses, went inside. The explosion had wrecked the cabin, tossing big logs all around. We found some parts of the bodies of the Kelly boys, with clothes sticking to them, and blood on the logs. The rest was under logs and dirt. We could see the big hole in the ground just under the boys' bunk, and we found a piece of fuse on a bush. It was clear how it had happened.

When the Kelly boys were asleep, this outlaw gang had sneaked up in the night and pushed a big charge of dynamite sticks under the floor where the bunk was, lit a fuse, and got away.

We rode home feeling sad, for the Kellys were fine boys. We heard later that the Kellys had made a great row over their loss when their horses were stolen, saying that they knew who was responsible for the loss, for they recognized the voice of Black as they heard him calling his men as the gang rode away in the dark. The Kellys threatened that they would get even with Black and his men.

Then another killing by the Black gang caused a lot of talk. A Jewish whisky drummer from a wholesale liquor house in Cheyenne wrote a letter to say that he was coming to our place, as he did twice a year, to take orders. This drummer was a good-natured fat Jew, who stood for the drinks, told us all the news of the outside world, and was quite a favorite with the boys. He never appeared and, while we were wondering what had become of him, news came that his body had been found on a sand bar down Elk River, with two bullet holes in him.

Later it leaked out that Black had shot him and thrown his body into the river. The drummer drove one horse, and in his buggy carried samples of liquor. Black offered the buggy for sale, so we felt sure that Black had killed him.

This Black was the leader of the outlaws who were stealing our horses and cattle. He was part Indian, short and powerful, with dark skin, black hair and eyes; a hard, cruel man, and a crack shot. He had been in jail for horse stealing, and had finally been run out of Wyoming. He had taken up a ranch at the east end of the bridge over Elk River about twenty miles east of us. Here he had built a saloon and dance hall where gambling and drinking went on all the time. Black was a smart politician, and stood in with the sheriff and the political crowd in power. He had a camp five miles up the river where he ran about three hundred head of fine horses. We all knew that most of these horses were stolen by his gang, as they were all branded stock and guarded day and night by as tough a bunch of man-killers as ever came to Colorado.

But the worst part of this Black outfit, and the phase that angered and disgusted all decent cattlemen, was the story of his domestic conditions. He was a widower with two daughters, about twenty and twenty-two years of age. These girls were really fine looking, with just enough of the Indian in them to give them a look of Italians—dark with the big black eyes—a coarse, bold beauty and very striking. By some strange whim of Black's, they had been brought up as boys; always dressed as cowboys, they were as good riders and ropers as any real cowboy. They were a rough couple, drank whisky and cursed like mule skinners. All this would have passed, as it was no one's business, but Black sold them out to anyone who could pay the price, and that made a scandal, even in such a rough and lawless country as this. Many talked of running all this Black family out of the country, but this was not easy, for hanging around he had some twenty men as bad as he was.

About this time I had a personal experience with Black. I was driving a bronco team in my buckboard, going to see a ranchman five miles east of Black's place, but I thought it was safe enough. I had no thought of any trouble, but as I trotted my team over the bridge, there was Black standing in the middle of the bridge, waving a revolver, cursing at me, and just drunk enough to be dangerous. Not another soul was in sight, for all were in the cabins at dinner. I was about half scared to death. I could not turn about and go back. The chills were running down my back, and as I thought of the Kelly boys blown up by this man, of the Jew drummer he had killed, I pulled my gun and pushed it under my right leg so as to have it handy. I called out, "I am in a hurry, Black! I have to see a patient," hoping he would let me by, but he stood right in the middle of the bridge, and I had to pull up. As I did so, Black pushed by the horses, came on my right side, putting his left hand on the seat to steady himself, and, leaning heavily over against me, he called me all the vile things he could think of, all the time waving his gun in his right hand and working himself up to the killing point.

I was so desperate that I almost drew up my gun to shoot him, but just then the door of the nearest cabin banged open and out came one of Black's daughters, who called out, "Dinner, Pa!" Black turned his head to answer her, and I had my chance! I had held my whip all the time, and as I lashed my team, they gave a spring forward. Black was twisted around, the hind wheel on that side hit his legs a jolt, and he was down on his back on the floor of the bridge. I was crouching down in front of the seat to avoid a shot, and pounding my broncos on the back at every jump. A turn in the road through some timber and I was out of sight. The sweat was running into my eyes, and I was shaking all over, but I laughed as I remembered old Black, mad and rolling in the dust. If he had meant only to frighten me, he had succeeded. I knew I had had a close call, and I kept looking back on the road to see if Black, in his black rage because of my stunt, had taken a horse and followed me.

After seeing my patient I did not have the courage to go back by the bridge. I knew that if Black was around he would force a fight, but I told myself I was not living up to my ideal of manhood. In a book I should have gone back and faced Black, but I backed out and took a longer way round. I worried over it, but when I reached home and told Squaw Charlie how ashamed I was, that tough Indian fighter gave me considerable comfort by saying, "Hell's fire, Doc! You done right. I'd 'a' done the same. That Black has his men around him and there's not a chance to make a getaway."

At last things came to a head. We had stood all outrages of these outlaws long enough. About twenty cattlemen got together at last, all men to be trusted, including the best people we had in the cattle business. We met at night in a private room back of the I.X.L. Saloon—no drinking, but all for serious business. The men came in one at a time, for spies were sure to be watching us to report to Black. The windows were covered with blankets; one small oil lamp flickered through dense tobacco smoke, bringing out the sanded floor and the unfailing spittoon. A table was in the middle of the room, rifles stacked in the corners—I can see this little room now as the men all crowded together around the table and spoke in whispers. Through the closed door we could hear the shouts of the tinhorn gamblers, "Make your bets, gentlemen," the shuffle of feet on the sanded floor, the giggling of the girls, and the same tune played on the old cracked piano. The boys were having a good time in the saloon; we were all used to it, and no one noticed it, for we were in deadly earnest. As one cowpuncher put it, "We run this range or the outlaws will. It is up to us."

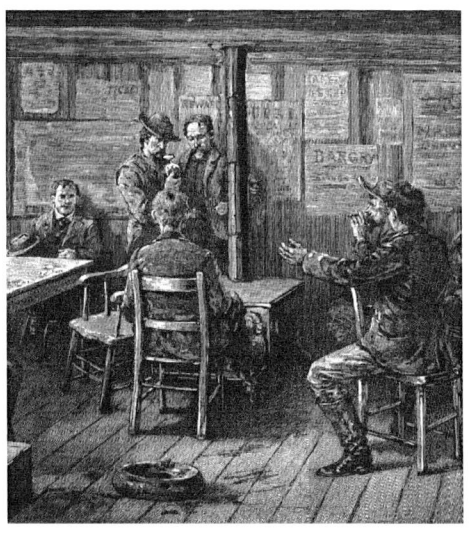

After some talk, we formed a vigilance committee to go and lynch Black—no need of a trial, we knew enough to hang him a dozen times over. All in order and according to rule, we elected a captain, decided that a small party, say of four men, was the best, the captain to select his men. Then all the rest went out, and I was going out with them, fondly believing that my duties would consist of acting in an advisory capacity only and that now I could go home to bed and safety and not be mixed up in any lynching party.

Then, to my surprise, the captain said, "Wait a minute, Doc!" I shut the door and joined the four men at the table. The captain, turning to me, said, "Doc, I been a-talking to the boys here, and we all want you to come along with us. You see, Doc, if we have any trouble and get shot, we want you handy to fix us up. Ain't that so, boys?"

"Sure," all the boys said, "we aim to have the doc go along."

So I just said, "All right, boys! Count on me," with a confidence I was far from feeling and with a sinking in the pit of my stomach that I was careful not to show by any outward signs.

As I glanced around at the faces in the dim light of the lamp, it suddenly struck me that by a strange freak of Fate, these four men were not only my best friends in the camp, but also that it was through my profession that I had come to know them so well. Of course the captain had chosen them for their courage, their skill with rifle and revolver, and their experience in scouting and fighting in a wild country. The captain selected was John Hall, a fine type of the old-time cowboy. Foreman of the D.O.D., a big cattle outfit, Hall had been bred to the wild West, had fought Indians when only a boy, knew cattle raising from hoof to horns, was a calm, quiet man of forty, and was loved by his men. I had cut out of his leg a piece of bone that had been bothering him for years, an old wound. "Sioux got me," he said, "down on the Sweetwater in 1865."

The man next to Hall around the table was a contrast to Hall. A boy of only twenty-two or twenty-three, Joe Blake was a buster for a ranch outfit, and it was said, the best rider in Colorado. For all his laughing face and his joking, Joe was a wonder with the revolver and, I fear, a natural killer. Anyway, Joe shot and killed a tinhorn gambler up at Aspen, and in the fight got his jaw smashed by a revolver bullet and lost a few teeth. I fed him with a rubber tube for some weeks.

The next man was out of the ordinary. Brown came from New York where he had known some of my people, had plenty of money, was a college man, and very much a gentleman. He had made a success of the cattle business and was owner of the largest and best ranch in our place. Brown, no doubt, did not at all relish this going on a lynching party, but felt it his duty. Twenty years before he had been a soldier in the Civil War; at that time he was noted for gallantry in action. A keen sportsman, he loved the Western life, was one of the best shots we had, and was a valuable man in any trouble. About forty years of age, a large strong man, always dignified and courteous to all, Brown was an outstanding figure among our settlers. He had been thrown by his horse near a wire fence on his ranch and dragged along the barbs of the fence and badly cut up. I managed to sew him up and, during his slow recovery, we became close friends.

The last man was called Squaw Charlie. He was a small, wiry, bowlegged specimen, whose history would make a wonderful book. Briefly told, both his parents were killed by Indians in a raid. He was adopted by the Indians and could talk with ease in several of their languages. At last he was taken by a trapper and taught to read and write, becoming a scout and interpreter with Custer and others. Keen and alert, his skill with a rifle was the admiration and talk of all the cowboys; a curious specimen, tough and without any nerves, he was, strange to say, reliable and honest in every detail. At this time he was breaking horses for an outfit to the west of us.

My interest in his curious history and his stories of his Indian childhood and battles with other Indians, drew us together. However, the main cause of our friendship came through an accident. He was riding what is called in cow land "a bad one," a bronco that went locoed or crazy, and in the mix-up Charlie was thrown against the logs of the breaking corral and his right shoulder was dislocated. There were some twelve punchers working on the ranch, and for two days the strongest ones had a pull on that arm, to draw it back into place, with no result except intense agony to Charlie. That poor victim, driven to desperate measures and with a shoulder swelling visibly after each pull, gave it out cold that he would shoot the next man who touched him; so one of the men rode in for me.

After battling with a snowstorm for forty-two miles over a rough trail, I was taken to the bunkhouse, and there was Squaw Charlie sitting up in a bunk, and looking as if murder would be a relief. I put him on his back on the hard dirt floor and, sitting at his right on the floor, facing him, I took off my right boot and put the heel of my foot into his right armpit. I grasped the lower part of his right arm and pulled it out along the floor at right angles to his body. All the boys were sitting in a ring around us to see the fun and to kid us along. I pulled his arm in a half circle down to his side, at the same time giving my right heel a kick into his armpit. There was a snap as the head of the bone jumped into the socket, a yell from Charlie, while the boys cried out, "Ain't Doc hell!" patting me on the back. I had not only reduced a dislocation, but I had also made a friend for life. These were the reasons why I knew these men around that table so well. It was all due to my profession.

Hall now told us his plan to capture Black. Every morning Black left his ranch on Elk River and rode along a trail by the river to his horse camp, some five miles away. He gave his orders to the men at the camp, looked at some of the horses, decided which ones to drive away to sell, all as if conducting a regular business. About halfway to this camp the trail passed over the top of a bare hill for one hundred yards or so, and right by the side of the trail there were three big rocks. Hall was to hide behind these rocks while it was still dark. The other men were to hide in the scrub oak fifty yards from the trail, and, as Black rode along the trail to the rocks, Hall was to challenge him to halt and throw his hands up. If Black showed any fight, Squaw Charlie from the scrub oak was to shoot him. No others were to fire. Black's men might be near and the others must be ready in case of trouble. As Hall frankly said, there was no use of taking any chances with a man like Black. If he would surrender, all right; if not, he would be shot from ambush, as one would kill an animal. It seemed like murder to me, but my friends were old Indian fighters and knew their business.

I went home to get my instruments and rifle, meeting the others about a mile out of town on the main road. It was midnight, with a clear sky and a new moon, enough light to travel by. I found all four waiting for me and, without a word, we followed Hall as he took an old game trail that wound back into the hills far from any ranch. We rode in single file, no one speaking, the figures in front of me looking like shadows. The silence was broken only by the sound of the ponies' feet on the soft trail, as we went along at the tireless fox trot of the bronco, climbing hills at a walk, fording streams when the horses snatched a few mouthfuls of water, through timber when the branches flew back and hit my face. The creaking of saddle leather, the tinkle of spurs, a horse coughing and being sworn at, were the only sounds for mile after mile. I lost my sense of direction, but Hall never wavered, as, quiet and stern as Fate, he held his way as if by instinct.

After hours, as it seemed to me, Hall stopped his horse in a thin grove of cottonwoods where just enough moonlight was

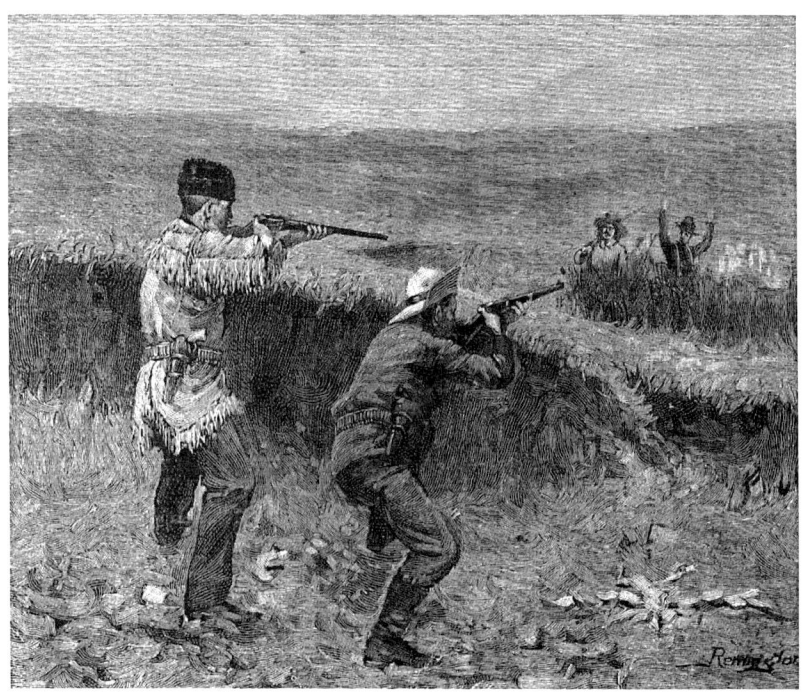

coming through the leaves to show me a vague outline of horses and men. Hall said, "You boys leave your horses with Doc and come with me; if Doc hears any shooting he's to come on with the horses." He pointed to a dark shadow about half a mile to the east. "That's the hill. The trail goes over the top right in front of you." All the men dismounted and gave me the lead ropes of their ponies. Brown, as he passed me his, said, "Good luck, Doctor, I wish I were in your boots." The men, carrying their Winchesters, vanished in the shadows.

 I was alone. The night breeze stirred the leaves of the cottonwoods overhead with a soft rustling, and I could see them quivering against the sky. The horses moved restlessly, pawed the ground, and tried to graze. I had trouble to keep their lead ropes all straight as they kept going around trees. I might have to make a dash for it at any time. I grew very nervous and lonely, and wondered what the boys were doing. I shivered as I thought of their work. At last gray light crept over the grove of trees and the prairie in front of me. I could see the horses around me, their breath looking like smoke in the cool air. The birds in the trees began to chatter and fly about. A coyote yapped in some timber behind us. The light grew stronger, and then the sunlight came over the hill. It was a glorious morning and, as I watched the fleecy clouds as they floated overhead all rosy against the deep blue sky, I wondered if Black was seeing them also. I looked again at the hill, still dark and in shadow, and then a bright streak of fire flashed out for a second on its dark side followed by the crack of a rifle. I felt sure the boys had been surprised and were fighting with the outlaws. I wondered that there were no more shots, but I must hurry, and I drove the spurs in, yelled at the other horses, pulled on the four lead ropes, and we were off in a bunch, slashing through small trees and galloping as if in a race across the little prairie and up the dark side of the hill.

 On top in the sunlight were the boys. I circled around them before I could stop. Each man ran to me and got his own horse. I got off and went over where Hall was bending above a figure on the ground. As I joined him he rolled the body over on its back, and there in the bright sunlight was the evil face of Black, those cruel black eyes that had stared into mine in anger so short a time ago now fixed in the unseeing stare of death at the blue sky. The mouth was twisted in a grin, showing the yellow teeth. His hat had fallen off, and the straight black hair lifted up and down in the breeze. My knees were shaking, and, fearing the boys would notice it, I knelt down by the body, unbuttoned the red woolen shirt and found the small dark hole of the .44 Winchester bullet just by the left nipple. Hall stood by and remarked in a quiet voice, "A good shot, Charlie, up hill against the light, and him a-rearing back so sudden." I looked at Charlie; for a moment his face lit up at the compliment, and then with a calm glance at the body, he cut a chew from his navy plug, tucked it into his mouth with fingers as steady as a rock, and pulled his horse around ready to mount.

I was told how it happened. When Hall had called to Black to stop, Black pulled his horse back, slung the rifle he was carrying to his shoulder to fire at Hall's voice coming from the rocks. Charlie, from the scrub oak, where all the time he had Black lined in his sight, fired. Black stiffened in the saddle and then slowly fell to the ground; one foot caught in the stirrup, and his horse circled around, kicking and bucking. Hall ran out and caught him.

Joe Blake now said, "Let's be going, Hall." Just then we heard the clatter of horses' hoofs on the trail coming up the hill. We all jumped behind our horses, rifles ready. Brown, who was near the edge and could see the trail, called out, "Don't shoot, boys! It's one of Black's girls!" And here she came, galloping like mad. Dressed like a cowboy, never giving us a glance, she jerked her bronco up short by the body of her father and sprang to the ground beside him. We stood as if frozen. This was awful! We braced ourselves for tears and reproaches, but nothing happened like that. This unnatural daughter was kneeling by her dead father, rapidly and with a fearful skill born of practice going through all his pockets for money. Finding only some plug tobacco and a knife, she rose to her feet and, with a fierce gesture of anger, threw these far from her. Then, to our disgust and horror, she commenced to kick the limp body, swearing and cursing at every kick, in an outburst of anger and spite that was terrible to see. Brown, white with emotion, muttered, "Hell! I can't stand this," and ran forward to stop her, but the girl was too quick for him; swinging around like a flash, she sprang on her horse and, in a whirl of dust, was gone down the trail. The rattle of hoofs on the stones of the rough trail faded and was gone.

We stood for a moment as if dreaming. Hall's voice saying "Come, boys" broke the spell. We all mounted. I was riding by Squaw Charlie. He looked back, stopped his horse, saying, "Wait a minute, Doc." I saw him run back where Black's big hat had fallen off, pick it up, go over to the body, and put it carefully over the face, then put a rock on the rim to keep it from blowing away. When he rejoined me he glanced at me as if embarrassed, and said, "It seems kinder more decent that-a-way, Doc." Good old Charlie! Such a curious mixture.

We rode hard on the back trail, as if anxious to be far away from all we had seen. Brown took a trail for his ranch, Hall another, Joe and Charlie loped off, and I rode into town alone. Strangely enough, no one seemed to know who killed Black. It never came out, so far as I know, even to this day. The effect on the outlaws was a stampede. They evidently thought we were far stronger than we were, and the country grew too hot for them. They scattered. The Black girls and some of the men drove off their horse herd. The cabins in some way caught fire and were burned down.

A year later I chanced to ride over the bridge. A quiet German family had pre-empted the ranch, built a new cabin. A wheat field covered the land, and a bunch of towheaded children laughed and played where the cards and whisky once held sway. I rode up the trail to the hill where Black was shot. A few bones were scattered among the rocks and sage bushes where the coyotes had dragged them, a ragged bit of red shirt fluttered in the wind from the top of a dead sage bush, mute evidence of the old order of crime and bloodshed now passed into history.

Chapter 20
Joe Bush and His Ride

That December afternoon was soft and mild for Colorado, but it was beginning to snow in big soft flakes that melted as they fell in the still air, and darkness was at hand. As I looked out of the window of my cabin I could see the lights of the little cow town beginning to glimmer here and there among the cabins. My room looked very cozy and comfortable with soft easy chairs, rugs, a German student lamp on the table, a shelf of books; and my open fire very bright and warm as it threw shadows among the deer heads on the wall and was reflected from my rifles in a rack below them.

I turned again to look at the snow, and was promising myself a long, comfortable evening with my books, when I heard the sound of a horse galloping on the bridge. I had built my bridge over a small creek that ran between the town and my cabin, for I had grown tired of splashing through the creek every time I went to town, about two hundred yards away. It was not much of a bridge; the floor boards were loose and noisy; but it was unique in one way, and that was that this noisy bridge acted as a kind of doorbell to my cabin, for, when a man rode over this private bridge of mine he was coming to see me, for the road came only to my cabin.

When I heard the clatter of hoofs on the bridge I knew not only that a visitor was coming, but more than this, I could tell how urgent the case might be. If the rider came merely to consult me about some simple illness of no great moment, I could hear the hoofs of his horse come tapping along the boards in a soft easy way at a slow fox trot; but when the call was an urgent one and the doctor was needed in a hurry, I could hear the hoofs of the bronco rattle the boards as, in a rush, he made two jumps of it. Then I knew there was really a serious case for the doctor, and since I was the only doctor for eighty miles around, probably I was in for a long, hard trip. This evening I heard the bronco make two jumps of it, and, when I reached the door and opened it meet the rider, there was "Shorty," a wrangler from the A-Bar-A Ranch twelve miles up the river.

Shorty was one of the silent kind of cowboys, and silently he swung off the saddle, leaving his bronco to stand in the snow and get his breath. Shorty beat the snow out of his hat and came into my room and, glancing anxiously around to see a safe place to spit his tobacco juice, at last used the fire to his evident relief. Shorty was not happy in a well-furnished home; he had lived too long in open camps, and it was only after some urging that he finally sat down on the extreme edge of one of my chairs—very carefully, as if this article of furniture might suddenly buck him off.

These minor points attended to in silence and dignity, Shorty, feeling more comfortable, at last gave me the message. He had been at dinner in the bunkhouse when a strange puncher had ridden up who was just skin and bone and so weak that one of the boys ran out and caught him as he was falling off his bronco. The boys carried him in and put him in a bunk. The foreman called out, "Say, Shorty, you ride down and tell Doc to come a-running or this sick bird will be a-dying on us!"

And Shorty had ridden down. He had told me all that he knew. I tried to get some details but failed. I could bar out childbirth, but that was about all, so I thanked Shorty, who left for town, anxious to have some whisky and to buck some game at the I. X. L. Saloon. I saddled up—no reading by my fire that night! Instead, I rode through the wet snow to the A-Bar-A. The dogs barked as I let down the bars at the big pasture, and Jake, the foreman, opened the door of the bunkhouse and called out, "That you, Doc?" As I dismounted in the path of light from the open door, Jake called out, "Some of you boys take the doctor's horse."

The bunkhouse of the A-Bar-A was quite different from the usual bunkhouse of that time, which was a dirty, mud-floored cabin used only for the men to sleep in at night, with things generally in a mess. But the A-Bar-A bunkhouse was a fine one, some twenty by sixty feet, made of big logs, with a dirt roof, but a board floor. Down the center was a long table. A kerosene lamp hung from the ridge log overhead. A fireplace was at one end, and at the other a big cookstove, where the darky cook was busy making bread; on one side were bunks against the wall, and on the other side, pegs from which hung saddles, bridles, ropes, slickers, and branding irons. It seemed very cozy and warm after the dark, stormy night outside. Some of the punchers were playing cards at the long table; others were mending saddles or ropes by the fire. As I knew them all I was soon shaking the snow from my clothes and sitting down with them. I asked Jake where my patient was, and he pointed to a little room near the cookstove, used for a storeroom. It had a bunk in it, and they had put the strange puncher in there where it was quiet.

It was interesting to me to see how the punchers took the arrival of this stranger. The old-time cowboy, as I knew him

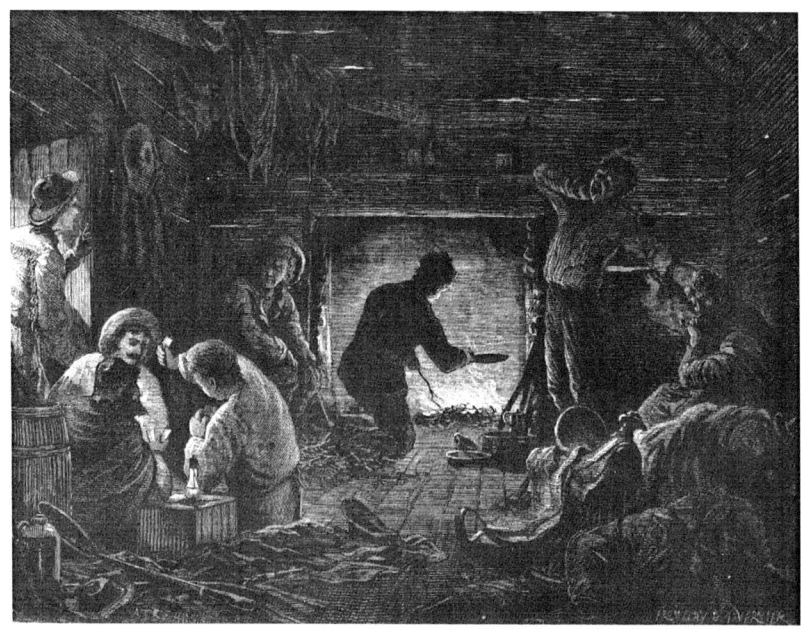

in Colorado, had a code of conduct quite as binding as that of any gentleman in civilization, and he held to it quite as strictly. This strange sick man was tenderly cared for, put to bed, his horse unsaddled, fed and watered as one of their own, and then, everything done, tiptoeing out very carefully, these cowpunchers left him alone.

There were some twelve punchers spending the winter at the A-Bar-A, eating and sleeping in the bunkhouse like one large family. You would imagine that some among them, seeing a stranger suddenly brought in so ill and wounded, would have asked him, "How did you get shot?" "What is your name and where do you come from?" But not one question was asked him, for such ill manners would have been considered very bad indeed. For six hours this stranger had lain silent in his bunk. The boys may have been curious about him, but true to their cowboy idea of good breeding, no one by look or word as much as hinted at any desire to know his history. Like Indians, they gave the stranger food, shelter, and rest, and if he told them his story, all right; if he kept silent, that was his business.

As I sat there among these rough, uncouth punchers, so cut off from the nice distinctions of civilized conduct, so used to violence and rough struggle with men and beasts, I could not help contrasting their tactful and kind consideration of this helpless man with the actions of a crowd in New York. While I was on the ambulance service for a big hospital, I would drive up to a crowd in the street, where a poor victim lay on the pavement, a crowd of the curious pushing and struggling over the prone form, shutting out all the air. I try in vain to make a little space to work—no use. The free show is too attractive—the pale face, the blood on the stones. A forest of legs hems him in. I shout and push, am laughed at; and then I whistle and call a policeman, who brutally beats about to create a spot for me to kneel and apply first aid. I prefer the cowboy and his savage ways. At least he is a gentleman at heart.

So I was not in the least surprised that no one knew this stranger's name, where he came from, or how he got shot; but it must not be supposed that these keen riders of the plains had not noted several things about this man and his outfit. In the first place, they all knew at once that he was a brother puncher, by a dozen signs on his belongings: the saddle was made in Pueblo; his rope was coiled properly in its strap below the horn; a cinch had been mended as only a cowboy with a knife and leather strings could do it. Then, his bronco had a vented brand from an outfit near Cheyenne, and another, a more recent one, used only by a cattle company in Old Mexico. A good cattleman in the old days knew every brand on the range, from the Rio Grande to the Canadian border, or seemed to. They also noted that his saddle blanket was Mexican and not Navajo, and that his spurs were the real old silver-mounted affairs, true Mexican. So they had a pretty good idea that this stranger had been "working below the border."

At last, when I was warm and comfortable and had had a word with all the punchers, most of whom were old friends, the foreman said we had better see this patient. We entered the little storeroom where, on a bunk, lay a boy of twenty-three, a shadow worn to skin and bone. His eyes sunken, hair long and tangled, clothes in rags, he was dirty, lousy, weak, with his left leg swollen, red, and discharging pus, and with a fearful smell of dead flesh. He was game and tried to smile as Jake put the lamp on the table and said, "Here's the doctor." I asked him no questions, but called in two of the boys. The cook heated water, and we washed and dressed a wound in the calf extending to the bone. I removed some bits of woolen cloth that had been carried into the wound, causing it to break out again.

One of the boys, without orders from me, dumped his bedroll on the floor near the bunk and announced, "I am night herding this stranger tonight." I heard him get up a dozen times during the night to give the patient a drink or to shift him to a more comfortable position. As a matter of course, the punchers took turns doing this service every night. It was a part of the code, and when you hinted that they were very kind, you were instantly told to "go to hell." Sentiment was not welcome.

In the morning the patient told me that his name was Joe Bush. He was in bad condition, with high fever, an infected wound, and starved to a shadow, so I stayed a week at the A-Bar-A Ranch, working over this boy. I tried to do some nursing, but the punchers would not hear of my doing it for a moment, and the gentle way these boys nursed this stranger was a wonder to me. One wrangler, of evil reputation as a killer, rode up to our little town every day and brought back a bottle of milk for Joe, as there were no milking cows at the ranch. At the end of a week my patient was well on the road to health, and anxious about his bronco; so the boys rounded the horse up and ran him through the big pasture where he could be seen by Joe, who was propped up in a chair near the window. This sight of his cow pony, now fat and strong, seemed to do Joe a lot of good, and he confided to me that he "set great store on that horse." He called him "Chuck-a-luck," and said, "Doc, that horse has as much sense as most humans."

Gradually I gained the confidence of the shy young puncher and, bit by bit, I had his story. He, of course, was quite unconscious that his story was at all unusual, and would have shut up for good if he had suspected that I was making notes about him on the side.

Joe Bush told me that he had been punching since he was a little shaver. His father was a cattleman up near Cheyenne, and with his father he had made the drive from Texas to Kansas, that long drive when in those early days the cowboys held the herd together for months, braving stampedes, hunger, thirst, hostile Indians, and cattle thieves; so this Joe Bush was a seasoned cattleman and fighter at an age when most boys were going to school. Shrunken and weak from his long ride, I could still see what a fine, strong specimen of manhood he must be at his best.

"You see, Doc," he said to me one day, "at the end of the last drive from Texas, our driver boss, Mat Williams, says to me, 'Joe, I got a chance to go down to Old Mexico. You see, some of them big cattlemen down there is having their stock run off by rustlers, and their Mexican cowboys ain't holding 'em back; so this big gun called a "don," who owns the stock and a ranch as big as outdoors, he writes the cattle association up here to pick out six cowboys and send 'em down to his ranch to fight rustlers. Wages is sure good, so I am going. How about your coming, Joe?' So I says, 'Mat, you count me in on that deal!'

"Well, Doc, the next thing I knowed, we had pulled our freight for the border, and I was riding for this Spanish outfit. Their hacienda was a big one, sure enough, and the *vaqueros* were all right to work with and could throw a rope with the best. And then the country seemed like home, just like Arizona, with greasewood and cactus a-growing everywhere, and horned toads and rattlesnakes. We were down Sonora way, only about mebby three hundred miles off the border. There was a Mexican town some six miles from the ranch, not much of a place, mud houses and all that, but there was some dandy Mex girls all right, and as for gambling! Well, those Mexicans just naturally took to it, and we sure painted that old town red a few times. Of course, we done some killing—going after some rustlers—and the old don was plenty proud of us, killing off the rustlers and cleaning up the country that-a-way. But I guess I played the fool all right, Doc, for I kinder felt my oats a bit, and got me a silver hatband and a red saddle blanket, and went into town a-looking for trouble, I guess, with my horse Chuck-a-luck dancing along down the street, and me a-bowing to the girls, and the men just looking hostile and mean enough to knife me. But I never cared, and played around with the girls, went to the dances, gambled all my money away, and got so lit up on their cactus brandy that I could hardly keep on my horse going home. Of course, the old drive boss kept a-telling me to quit all this foolishness or I'd get a knife in my ribs some night, but I only laughed, as kids will, being that foolish and stuck on myself, and then one night I met the little Mexican girl, and got in bad. No matter about her name. I met her at the *Fiesta*. There was the usual old woman night herding her, but I managed to see her alone, and say, Doc, she was a dandy, as pretty as a new chuck wagon! Her big black eyes was snapping, and she had a rose stuck over one ear. I fell hard, sure enough. I never knowed her folks, or where she come from. I was plenty innocent, all right, never suspicioned anything—just went ahead and made hot love to her at the first jump out of the box, and she kinder took a fancy to me. Anyhow, I laid low and said nothing to the boys, and the girl kept telling me to be careful, not to be seen with her or there would be hell to pay. So I moseyed around on the sly and rented a little mud house on a back street, and only met her there after dark when the people around were asleep. She taught me how to play the guitar and sing in Spanish, a sort of cowpen Spanish, but good enough. We only met about two nights a week. I was nighthawking for the ranch outfit some nights and could not get away. Well, everything went on fine. I gave the girl quite a lot of presents, and was that soft and easy it most makes me sick to think of it now, and she a-stuffing the pack agin me all the time!"

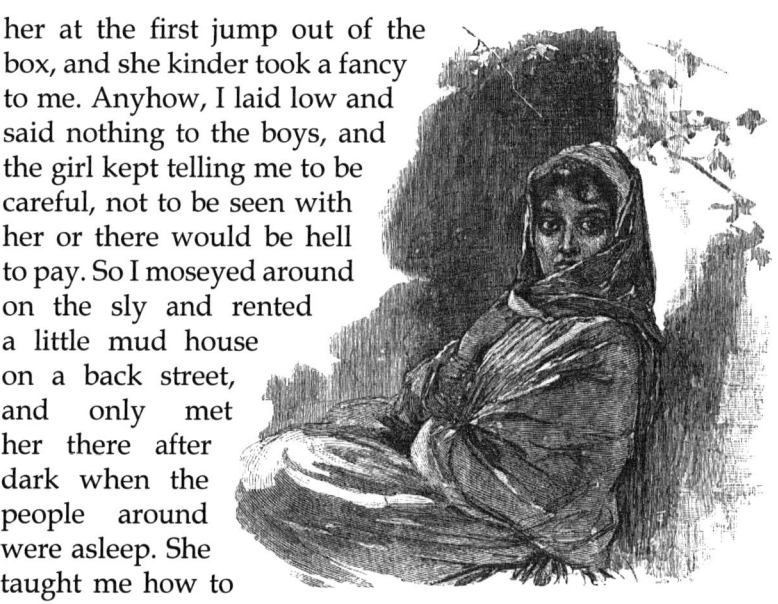

 I fear that Joe was quite true to type, and I can picture this good-looking young puncher, all arrayed in his best, in the barbaric splendor of silver hatband, red handkerchief around his neck, fringed chaps, big spurs, two revolvers, his fair hair waving over his tanned face, his blue eyes dancing with fun, riding proudly among the sullen, hostile Mexicans. No doubt he lorded it over them, as he flirted with their girls with a humorous, devil-may-care aspect, ready to make love or to fight at the drop of the hat, and doubtless driving the Mexican men into a frenzy of jealousy and rage at this hated gringo. He did not go without warning, for his friend, the drive boss, more than once warned him, saying with much truth, "Say, son, if you go a-mixing about with these greasers of nights, you sure will stop a knife."

But Joe, afraid of nothing, merely laughed and went his way, as youth generally does. Things move rapidly below the border. I suspect that this Mexican girl was a sly one, and Joe, for all his experience as an Indian fighter, bronco buster, and wilderness rider, was a singularly simple child when it came to the female of the species. All he knew was good women and bad women, and very little of either, so he was taken in; he swallowed bait and hook, as many a good man before him. Morals seem to have played very little part in this rough romance. I suppose Joe never gave it a thought that he was living over a volcano during his visits to this little cabin where he met the Mexican girl, who was sly enough to conceal from Joe that she had, for some time, been the favorite mistress of the chief of police. Quite happy and contented, the candle giving a dim light in the interior where Joe played the guitar and sang, the girl laughing at his clumsy efforts and his funny Spanish accent, the narrow street outside quite dark and silent, with its open sewer in the middle giving off its vile vapors in the warm air, they thought themselves alone, and were certain that no one knew of these stolen midnight hours, for Joe always left before daylight and was at the ranch for work as usual.

"Well, Doc," Joe continued, "I kinder sensed I was looking for trouble in taking up with that Mexican girl, but you know how it is, never seeing no white woman, and she such a pretty piece. I guess she locoed me at the time. I kept pretty dark about it all, as I told you, and thought I was smart and no one knew nothing about it. I never knowed her folks or anything, or where she lived, and never asked her. I guess she'd a lied to me if I had. We could only meet at night, as I said, so I put my horse in a corral and walked to the house—not much of a place, just a one-room shack with a table, two chairs, and a bed; a dirty mud floor, with the one door opening on the narrow street, but it was quiet and no one minded us, for the neighbors was all asleep long ago, and when she come in, her eyes laughing and her white teeth a-shining, I just forgot all about the mud shack. We were in Paradise! That girl lit it all up as if it was gold. Strange, what a damn fool a man can be sometimes, when a girl gets her cinch on him.

"Well, everything went on lovely for quite a time. I know that people were a-watching us and spying on us, and reporting to the police, and trouble was a-hatching for me; but I didn't worry none, just careless I guess. Anyhow, there we was one night, me a-sitting on the bed and she a-showing me how to play the guitar she brought along. She was a-looking like a thousand dollars, and me a-sitting there a-looking at her like a sick calf, when all of a sudden someone was a-knocking at the door and hollering 'Open in the name of the law!' I was for going to open the door myself, but the girl she grabs my arm and whispers to me, 'Let me talk!' She was fierce about it. I buckled on my gun and jumped in a corner. The girl blows out the candle and opens the door wide. There was a small crowd around the door holding torches, and people kept running up to see the fuss. A kind of red light lit up the room, and in walked the chief of police and his deputy, both armed and ugly looking.

"The chief was a little, dark, fat Mexican, marked with smallpox, who never saw me or took no notice of me anyhow, and then the girl let out a string of talk at the chief, making excuses, I guess. She talked so fast I could not understand it all. The chief flew into a rage and caught the girl by one shoulder. She twisted away, and the dress tore loose. Then this skunk of a chief he grabbed the girl's hair and commenced to slap her face. Well, Doc, I just got mad, forgot about my gun, and in two jumps I was over by the chief. I gave him a slam on the jaw. He fell against the wall, his mouth bleeding, and looking like a timber wolf. He pulled his gun. I had no time to draw, so I shot from the hip. He gave a grunt and slumped down on the floor. He kicked a few times and lay still.

"Then behind me the deputy shot his old carbine, and the slugs caught me in the leg. I fell against the table. The girl ran out the door a-screaming, and the deputy dropped his carbine and followed her. I was choking and coughing in all the black powder smoke in the room, so I hopped to the door. The crowd had run away, and I saw the deputy a-running down the street, just turning the next corner. I was mad all through. I just throwed my gun down on the deputy and let him have it. At the shot he threw his arms up and fell against the wall of a house, then slid into the gutter and lay there, his big hat a-rolling on the rim down the street like a cart wheel. Then I looked around, and there was the police all around me, a-holding their carbines not two feet away from my head. Fighting wasn't no use. I called out in Spanish, 'I surrender,' and threw down my gun, and the next moment a lasso was around my neck. I was jerked into the street and tied, hand and foot; the police grabbed me, half carrying and half dragging me along. The crowd yelled 'Kill the gringo!' and kept a-coming, but we turned a corner, and there was the jail, a small stone building. Someone unlocked the door, and throwing me in, the police ran in after me, and slammed and bolted the big door. The stones rattled on the door. We were just in time, and the stones sounded like a drum in the small cell."

The sounds outside gradually grew less as the crowd melted away. A guard struck a light, and Joe could see his ragged captors sitting on the floor against the wall, their big hats casting a shadow over their dark, evil faces. All lit cigarettes and talked together. Joe could see the dark and dirty stones of the walls, the floor littered with the filth of ages, the beams of the smoke-darkened ceiling festooned with huge, dusty cobwebs waving back and forth in the air from a grating in one wall. It was bare — not even a box to sit on. Joe had seen the jail before. It was a small stone building, said to be a hundred years old. He had ridden around it and seen at one end the stone wall splashed with lead from the bullets that had killed a group of prisoners one morning as they stood bound and helpless in the chill dawn, and Joe had ridden away, glad to be out of sight of the evil place.

"I tell you, Doc," Joe resumed later, "I was sure having one hell of a time. These greasers had hog-tied me, up and down, so I could hardly breathe, my leg was a-hurting me something fierce, and my mouth was dry and full of dust. I wasn't a-whining none, but I was as near crazy with thirst as a man can get, so I calls out in Spanish for a drink of water. One of these bucks setting against the wall just got up with a grunt, and I thought for sure I was a-going to have a drink all right, but I might have knowed better, as this greaser just come over to where I was laying helpless as a baby and gave me a kick in the ribs that near finished me, I being that weak. Then all the other greasers laughed and seemed to think it a good joke.

Pretty soon one greaser got up and looked out of the door. All was quiet outside, and, telling the others to come on, they all went out and locked the door on me. I was sure I was going to be shot at sunup, but I was that bad I only hoped it would come quick, and the only reason I was not shot, I figure, was that the Spaniard who owned the ranch where we were working had told the police to keep out of trouble with the American cowboys, or any rate not to do any shooting without a trial."

All had gone through the big door, the key was turned, and Joe was alone in his misery. He twisted and turned, but the ropes held him helpless; the little fire of brush in the middle of the dirt floor sank into a few embers, and the room, now dark, grew chill as a tomb. As the night wore on, Joe could hear the guards making their rounds outside the jail. The bells from a church clanged out the weary hours with a harsh note, and Joe wondered why they had not shot him. He slept at times, a kind of stupor, and daylight at last sent a faint light through the grating in the wall; voices were heard outside, the big door opened, and sunlight and fresh air came in.

A man entered and stood over him. A kind voice gave orders to the guards. The ropes binding his body so tightly were taken off, and the man knelt down by him, telling Joe that he was a doctor sent by his friends. Joe tried to speak, but no sound came, for his tongue and mouth were swollen and dry. This man gave orders. A can was put to Joe's lips, the doctor holding up his head with one arm. Never had a drink seemed so fine. This physician was well dressed and seemed a man of education. For a week he dressed Joe's wound and gave him every care, but nothing made him talk. To all the questions that Joe asked he smiled and shook his head.

Joe now had some straw to lie on, and an old woman brought him some food every day. No other prisoners arrived. Joe's splendid health came to the rescue, and he was gaining strength every hour. He was hardened to discomfort. His young body had never known anything but the rough life of a puncher — sleeping on the ground, wet and cold, going hungry, often dirty and lousy for weeks; so the jail was not so much of a change. Physically he did not mind; it was the confinement that made his punishment. Living as he had all his life out in the open, free as a bird, with nothing but plain and mountain around him and the blue sky overhead, the dark walls of the jail seemed to close in on him, making him like a tiger from the wilds, caught and put in a cage. There were times when, he confessed to me, he thought he should go crazy. There was nothing to do but to wait and look at the stones, watch the spiders in the webs overhead, and see the lights from the small grated window slowly make a path across the heaps of refuse on the mud floor.

After a life filled with adventure and change, it was awful to Joe, as if he were buried alive in a stone box. In his boyish, bashful way, he told me that a change came over him. He had never really thought about his life before, and now, in the silence and loneliness of this dark prison, he made up his mind that if he ever did escape, he would first try to educate himself and then strike out for something better. He saw as never before that a puncher's life was all right for a time, but it led to nothing, and, as he said, "I saw myself an old man, full of whisky, just riding the fences, a broken-down cowboy, not knowing anything, not saving anything; and gosh! Doc, I just said to myself, 'Joe, you damn fool, if you ever get out of this place you git a move on and do something.'"

He wondered what his friends at the ranch were doing, and if there were a chance of escape, but he felt there was little hope. He regretted now that he had killed the deputy. Two greasers at one time! No, he felt in his bones that he was sure to be shot. No mercy now! Well, he would "die game and like an American cowboy, anyway, and be damned to them!"

On the twenty-first day, the old woman came hobbling in as usual, and Joe, as always, joked and teased her. This morning she came closer and whispered "Tonight," and without another word hobbled out, and the guards shut the door. All that day Joe limped on his wounded leg up and down the uneven dirt floor of his prison, wondering what the old Mexican woman had meant by "Tonight." Was it a warning that he was going to be shot, or were the boys at the ranch coming to get him out? He did not worry much about the shooting. If he were to be shot, well, "Let her go;" he had been in danger so often that he was a bit of a fatalist. However, the boys coming to break the jail and set him free did make his heart beat faster. He tried to imagine how they would do it, and, being young and a man of violent action, could only think of his cowboy pals as arriving with a rush of broncos, flashing guns, and wild yells, surrounding the jail, breaking in the door, and killing the Mexicans. All keyed up as he was by the thought of freedom and how it would feel once more to lope across the prairie on his favorite horse, Chuck-a-luck, with only the sky line around and the cool, pure air in his face, the waiting was weary work.

Darkness settled down, the church bells rang out the hours, and there were other sounds coming faintly through the tilted grating—sounds of laughter, music, shouts of a crowd making merry, girls running past the jail, giggling at the guards, asking them to go to the dance. Joe knew that there was a big *Fiesta* going on—some Saint's day, or holiday. At midnight Joe began

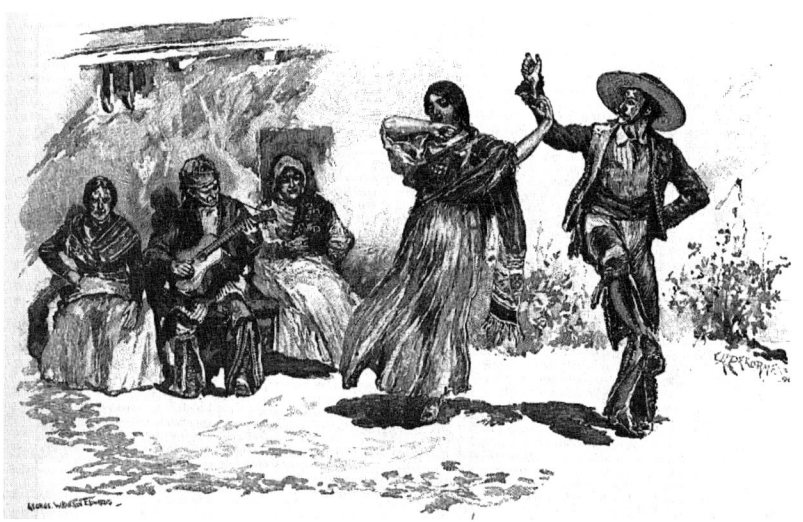

to lose courage. Were the boys coming? Then he heard horses, and men talking in whispers outside the jail door. With his ear to the door Joe tried to listen, to hear, and, for a moment, he thought that, after all, they were collecting outside to drag him out and shoot him during the confusion of the *Fiesta*. It looked like it. They were quiet. At last the door was unlocked, a head pushed itself in, and a voice that Joe knew as that of one of the boys, said in a whisper, "Come, Joe."

How his heart bounded with relief! He pushed through the door and was outside. He saw dark shadows of men and horses; a hand guided his limping footsteps to a horse, and, as he was helped into the saddle, the horse gave a soft nicker of remembrance. Joe, to his delight, knew that he was once more on his faithful friend and companion—his cow pony, Chuck-a-luck.

A voice in his ear in a husky whisper said, "We boys knowed you was a-going to be shot at sunup. Head north and keep a-going. Grub's rolled up in your slicker. Your guns and rifle is slung on the horse. Good luck, son!" and Joe, without a word, but with a thankful heart, was riding at a lope through the dirty little street, by cabins and shacks, past some ranches, and then in the open country, amid silence, and the stars shining down from a clear sky. Free, and a real horse under him!

At daylight he rode up a canyon he had noted in driving cattle, and lay hidden all day. There was water to be had by digging in the dry creek bed. Joe took off all his torn and dirty clothes and buried them, as he found a complete outfit rolled up in his slicker behind the saddle. Certainly the boys had been thoughtful about his comfort; not only had they given him his horse, the best he had ever owned, but also his own stock saddle, halter and rope, his two Colts and his Winchester, extra cartridges, and a full line of cowboy's clothes, from Stetson hat to spurs, also several pounds of dried beef, and some cakes. He felt like a prince as he "holed up" in that box canyon, and rubbed himself all over in the hot sand, while his pony ate the grass that grew in patches near the damp creek bed.

The next night he made north again and guessed that he must have crossed the border into the United States sometime near midnight. It was slow going, but he was skilled in all wilderness lore from his childhood, and could see the dark outline of mountains to guide him even in starlight.

For many days he pushed north through Arizona. He was soon out of food, but on a timbered mesa he shot a young buck, made a camp, and jerked the meat in the sun over the smoke of his campfire. He thought of riding into some ranch, but feared that the news of his escape was known and that there was a reward out for his capture, from the Mexican government. He realized later that there was no fear of this, but he felt safer in avoiding people, and he struck through a wild country. Once he saw a war party of Indians come out over a mesa about half a mile away, but he doubled back into the mountains and avoided them. The nights grew colder, and he could not sleep, for he feared to start a fire and sleep by it. He got some sleep during the day, and then the country got bare and treeless, and game was very scarce, for the deer had all gone down to the lower valleys. He snared rabbits, but he was often without food all day. After he reached Colorado his wounded leg began to give him trouble. It swelled, and he suffered every night from pain and chills. He now traveled by daylight, but he could not hunt afoot, for walking through the brush and over the uneven ground gave him intense pain. The wound opened up, swelling and turning black, and he knew it was in a bad way.

"Doc," he explained, "I was burning up with fever and shaking like I had the chills, and then a funny thing happened. I got kind of locoed, like I'd seen a horse that has eaten a loco weed. I kinder lost my sense, and all I could think of was them Mexicans hunting me. I hid out and never dared see no one; I would fall asleep at night and have a dream, always the same one. I was back in that old stinking jail, and them greasers tying my arms and putting me up against that stone wall outside. I could feel the cold stones against my back, and the greasers pointing their carbines at me, and then came the word to fire! Then I woke up with a start and a yell, all shivering and sweating, and old Chuck-a-luck would snort and pull on his picket rope, thinking there was Indians a-coming, I guess, and I was so weak I just lay there a-shaking."

One day he topped a mesa and looked down into a valley, so weak he could hardly stay in the saddle, and there in the valley was a fine ranch with horses and cattle. He could hear voices rising through the still air; smoke was coming out of the pipe of the big bunkhouse, and a smell of bacon cooking was wafted up to him among the pines on the hilltop. The cook came out and yelled, "Come a-running, boys." It was all so natural to him that he felt a surge of homesickness after the misery and loneliness of his long trip. He yearned for human beings; and the sight of this ranch, with the smell of cooking and the sound of horses, of men, so moved him that something seemed to snap in his brain; in a moment all the fear and delusions of capture vanished. He was sane again, and turning Chuck-a-luck downhill, rode off the mesa, through the big pasture, and up to the bunkhouse where, as I have told, he fell into the arms of one of the boys, and came to in a bunk, too feeble to talk.

I left Joe gaining every day, and his wound healing nicely. About a week later I rode up to the A-Bar-A to see how he was getting along. He was putting on flesh, and the change was wonderful to see. His splendid physique and the open-air life were beginning to tell in his favor. I found him sitting in front of the bunkhouse with a smile of delight on his face. He was watching his cow pony, Chuck-a-luck, as with a bunch of broncos of the horse herd, he was being raced past him by Frank Walker, the wrangler, to show Joe how well his horse was looking. Joe, pride in his voice, was saying, "Ain't he a dandy, Doc?" and I quite agreed with him. Chuck-a-luck was better bred than most broncos, and had a beautiful build as he loped past us, his head up, mane and tail flying. When Joe had limped into the house and no one was around, he said, "Doc, you sure have been a friend to me, and I ain't got a cent to pay you with, but if I have any luck I surely will pay you sometime."

I left the cattle country and settled down to a practice in one of Colorado's cities. Ten years passed. I had forgotten all about Joe Bush and his ride, when one day on my way to see patients at the hospital, I was stopped in the street by a very dignified man of about thirty-five, dressed in good taste, with a fine figure, tall and active. I gave the lines to my man, as my team was jumpy, and joined this stranger on the sidewalk. He laughed and said, "I bet you don't know me! Well, I am that Joe Bush you came to see at the A-Bar-A, shot in the leg."

I was glad to see the man again, and asked him to come up to the club. "No, Doc, I must be moving; have to catch a train for Leadville in half an hour. I am doing well in the mining game. Got out of cattle in the slump of 1885. Now, Doc, here's a hundred dollars, and I been looking for you ever since I made my strike. So long!" and he was hurrying for his train. For a moment I stood dazed, holding the roll of bills in my hand, and the old life came before me like a moving picture—the long rides, the danger, the dust, the bawling of calves, the hard riding, and the swearing, shooting punchers, laughing and carefree, who would kill you for an insult, and pay a forgotten debt, ten years old.

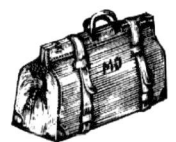

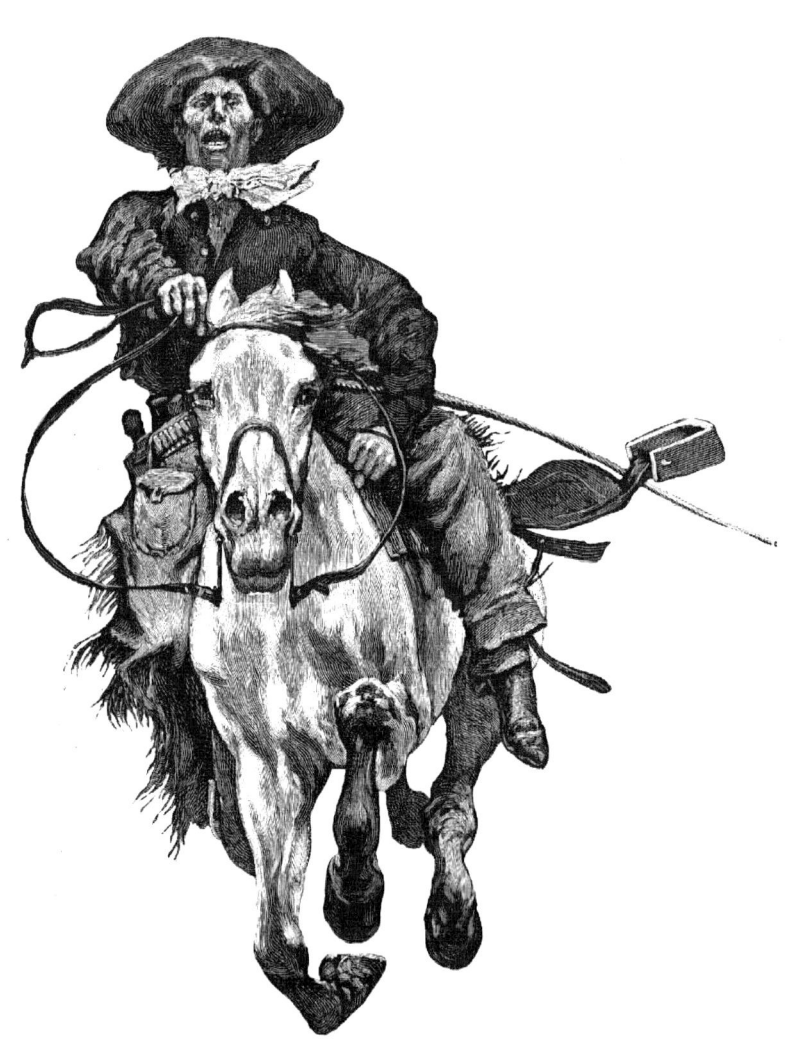